The Complete Mall Walker's Handbook

Walking for Fun and Fitness

The Complete

Mall Walker's Handbook

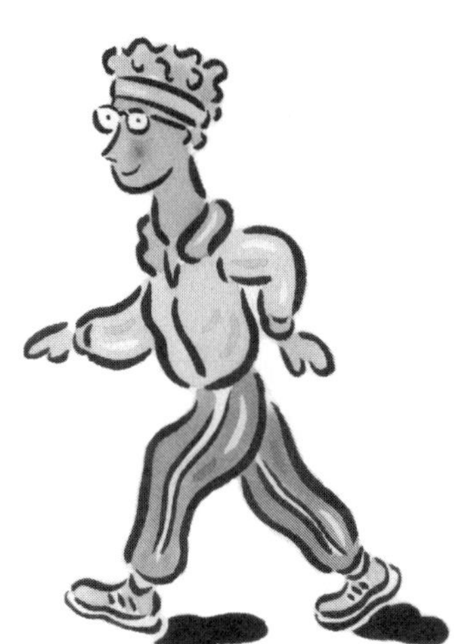

Walking for Fun and Fitness

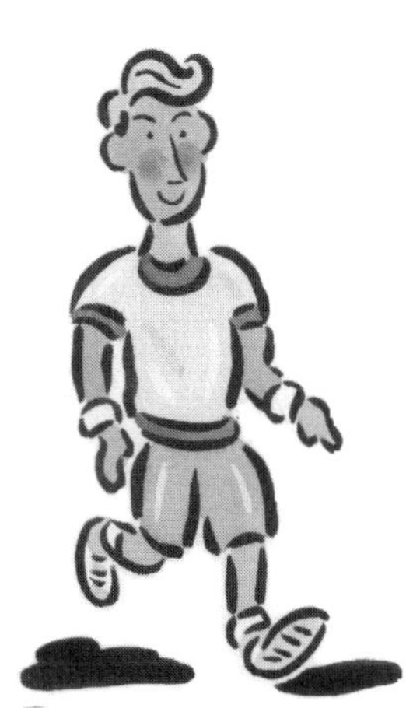

by John H. Bland, M.D.
with Jenna Colby, R.D., L.D.

Fairview Press
Minneapolis

Published by Fairview Press, 2450 Riverside Avenue, Minneapolis, MN 55454.

Library of Congress Cataloging-in-Publication Data

Bland, John H. (John Hardesty), 1917–

The complete mall walker's handbook : walking for fun and fitness / by John Bland, with Jenna Colby.

p. cm.

ISBN 1-57749-042-8 (alk. paper)

1. Fitness walking. I. Colby, Jenna. II. Title.

RA781.65.B575 1999 98-39713

613.7'146—DC21 CIP

First Printing: September 1999

Printed in the United States of America

03 02 01 00 99 7 6 5 4 3 2 1

Cover: *Cover Design by Laurie Ingram Duren™*

Illustrations: Miles Parnell

The Activity Pyramid and *The Activity Pyramid for People Over 60* reprinted with permission of Park Nicollet HealthSource® Institute for Research and Education.

The Food Pyramid for People Over 70 reprinted with permission of Tufts University School of Nutrition Science and Policy.

Publisher's Note: Fairview Press publications, including *The Complete Mall Walker's Handbook,* do not necessarily reflect the philosophy of Fairview Health Services.

For a free current catalog of Fairview Press titles, please call toll-free 1-800-544-8207. Or visit our website at *www.Press.Fairview.org.*

Acknowledgments

Books don't just happen! A good book—and this is a good book—requires the loving sacrifice of many people: family, colleagues, editors, teachers, reviewers, and, yes, patients.

I am indebted to Linda Mendenhall Bland—my editor, daughter, and best friend—for skillfully editing and imposing literary felicity on the finished manuscript. Thanks also to Dan Verdick for the very idea of the *The Complete Mall Walker's Handbook,* and to Lane Stiles and Jenna Colby for putting the original manuscript in such excellent working form.

The old musician's joke: How do you get to Carnegie Hall? PRACTICE! PRACTICE! PRACTICE! The simple truth: The hardest workers are the best performers. Walking is clearly the best of all exercises—no equipment required! So PRACTICE WALKING and overcome the decline of aging.

John H. Bland, M.D.

Thank you to my loving husband for his patience and kindness … and for being my lifetime companion.

And to my family, who has always been loving, supportive, and a great inspiration for exercise.

Special thanks to Fairview Press, ACCUSPLIT Inc., Park Nicollet HealthSource, Tufts University, Mall of America mall walkers, and everyone who took time to share with me what they enjoy about exercise.

Jenna Colby, R.D., L.D

Contents

Introduction

"I will tell you what I have learned about myself. For me, a long five- or six-mile walk helps. And one must go alone and every day."

BRENDA UELAND

Writer Brenda Ueland believed that walking every day was the key to clearing her mind, spending time by herself, and staying healthy and fit. Perhaps walking was also the key to her longevity—she lived until age ninety-four. She knew what many other people have discovered: A regular program of walking can yield significant physical and psychological benefits at any age.

Experts believe that walking regularly is a great way to condition your heart and lungs, improve circulation, reduce blood pressure, burn calories, and keep weight down. Walking also lessens stress and tension and sharpens your thinking. Many walkers have a positive self-image and a good outlook on life.

Why Walk?

The easy answer is "to get from place to place." You take thousands of steps each day, whether you're at home, at work, or out and about. The good news is walking can be more than just a way to get from point A to point B: You can walk your way to fitness and better health.

Research has shown that simply adding steps to your day can make you healthier. For example, you could take the stairs instead of the elevator, head to the grocery store or coffee shop on foot instead of by car, or park farther away from your destination so you have to walk a little longer than usual. All these activities add up to extra steps. You can reap even more rewards when you take your routine a step further by *briskly* walking for an extended period (anywhere from twenty minutes to an hour, depending on your fitness level) several times per week.

In 1996, the Surgeon General reported that Americans should do at least thirty minutes of physical activity on most days of the week—and preferably every day of the week. According to the Surgeon General, regular physical activity (along with a healthy diet) can improve your overall health and may reduce your risk of heart disease and some forms of cancer. Physical activity can include everything from swimming to dancing to . . . walking.

People all over the country are now walking to improve their fitness level and overall health (physical and mental). Is it really that easy? Yes. You don't have to belong to a health club or hire a personal trainer to get fit. Walking—in your neighborhood, on local paths or trails, or at the mall—is a great way to exercise and improve your health.

The wonderful thing about walking is that people of all ages and activity levels can do it. Walking doesn't require training, athletic skill, or special equipment (other than a good pair of shoes). Walking can be invigorating and fun on some days, calm and peaceful on others—*you* set the pace. Best of all, it's never too late to begin increasing your physical activity by walking: You can walk in your forties, sixties, eighties . . . or when you're over 100!

Why MALL Walk?

Although many mall walkers are senior citizens or people who have started a walking program following doctor's orders, anyone can mall walk for fun and fitness. Health experts promote mall walking because it's a convenient and easy way to exercise. Here are a few more good reasons to mall walk:

- **You don't have to worry about the weather.** When it's raining, snowing, or 98 degrees outside, you're sure to find better "weather" inside the mall. Malls are heated or air-conditioned (depending on the outdoor climate), so you'll be more comfortable during your exercise routine. You can mall walk rain or shine.
- **The terrain is smooth and even.** You don't have to be concerned about puddles, ice, mud, or hills—or fight the traffic of bicyclists, in-line skaters, and skateboarders. (This is especially good news if you have sore knees, arthritis, or other health concerns.)
- **It's safe.** Most malls are secure, well-lit, and full of people, and you don't have to consider the dangers of walking alone on an outdoor path. (*Bonus:* If you're traveling and don't know an area very well, you can usually rely on the local mall to be a reasonably safe—and free—place to exercise.)
- **It's social.** Mall walking is even more fun with a friend or loved one because you can walk and talk at the same time (and stop for a healthy snack afterward). If you mall walk on a regular basis, you'll probably see the same crowd certain days of the week. Because you have something in common, it's easy to strike up a conversation and get to know other mall walkers. In fact, some mall-walking groups become close and get together socially outside the mall.

Mall walking is a good fitness activity at any age, but if you're in your forties or fifties, mall walking can also serve as a way to control your weight and safeguard your health. If you're in your sixties, seventies, or eighties, mall walking on a regular basis can help you feel younger, more energetic, and more social. This type of exercise may even decrease your risk of serious illness and increase your life expectancy.

"Mall walking is fantastic! Exercise is only part of it . . . the bigger part is the social atmosphere. It allows a husband and wife one hour of uninterrupted conversation. Just get out and do it. People at the mall are like family. The scenery is great all year round. I suggest walking before the stores open—it's much cheaper."

ERNIE

How to Use This Book

Whether you're into mall walking for the health or social benefits (or both), this book can help you make the most of your mall-walking routine. You'll learn about the importance of exercise at any age, why it's crucial to stretch and stay limber, and how to start mall walking—and stick with it! You'll even find tips on starting a mall-walking program if your local mall doesn't have one already.

You'll also find suggestions for eating right, which goes hand-in-hand with getting in shape and taking charge of your health. We offer the basics on following a nutritious eating plan that focuses on the five food groups. Our goal is to help you make the right food choices—not put you on a diet. The key is moderation and a commitment to taking care of yourself from head to toe.

You can read this book from start to finish or dip in anywhere to find the information you're looking for. Throughout, you'll read testimonials from mall walkers who love the results they're getting—maybe they'll inspire you to head to the mall yourself. We've also included fascinating facts about walkers and surprising trivia about malls—we hope these will bring a smile to your face and help you remember that mall walking is FUN!

"I'm fifty-one. I've been running or walking vigorously since I was a freshman in college. That has been over thirty years now. My weight is the same as when I was a freshman in college, and I feel great. Now I'm mall walking. I plan to continue with my program because of how good I feel."

RON

1 Why is Exercise Important?

"So many people spend their health gaining wealth, and then have to spend their wealth to regain their health."
A. J. REB MATERI

"I don't have time to work out."
"I've never been in shape, so why bother exercising now?"
"After work, I'm too exhausted to think about exercise."
"I have better things to do."

Do any of these excuses sound familiar?

It's easy to get into the habit of saying you're too busy to exercise (or too tired, or too out of shape). Instead of telling yourself why you *shouldn't* exercise, think about all the good reasons why you *should.* Regular physical activity makes you stronger, leaner, healthier, and more fit. You'll feel better and look better. So it's time to put all the old excuses to rest!

Begin to think of exercise as something you do without question—like brushing your teeth. If your schedule is hectic, you can work out first thing in the morning (rise a half hour earlier than usual), during your lunch hour, or late in the evening. If you're tired, keep in mind that physical activity speeds up your heart rate and gets your blood pumping—a workout may be just what you need to feel refreshed and alert. And if you're feeling out of shape, remember that exercise is the best way to get fit. Once you start, you'll be on your way to feeling your best.

DID YOU KNOW . . .

Tired when you wake up? You may be walking more than you think. Sleepwalking is a harmless and not uncommon walking habit. It's most likely to occur when you're worried or tense, and may lead you to walk around your bedroom, turn lights on, and even get dressed or undressed. Episodes of sleepwalking may last 5–20 minutes, and they're more likely to occur early in the evening, about two hours after bedtime, and during deep slumber. Contrary to popular myth, it doesn't harm a sleepwalker to be awakened. (If you find yourself among the ranks of night crawlers, just think of it as a way to add an extra entry in your daily fitness log.)

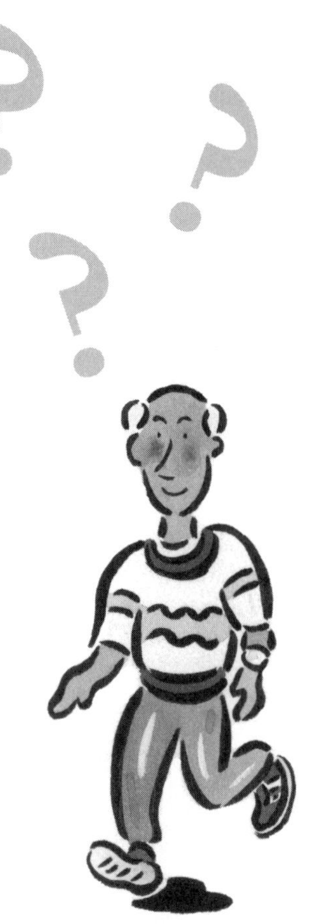

Amazing Walkers

Walk for the Health of It

"Walk for the Health of It" was the name of Robert Sweetgall's personal trek through America's 50 states—a challenge designed to spread the word about the health benefits of walking. On September 7, 1984, Sweetgall set out on what would be a journey of 11,600 miles—braving blizzards, heavy rains, rough winds, and blazing sun. The self-proclaimed "fitness salesman" teamed up with doctors who monitored his progress every step of the way. Millions of steps later, he helped prove what walking enthusiasts had long suspected: Without a doubt, walking helps your heart and improves your health.

Ten Great Reasons to Exercise

Whether you're considering getting in shape, just starting an exercise program, or setting new fitness goals for yourself, motivation is the key to your success. Whenever you need a boost, consider these ten reasons for getting—and staying—fit.

1. Exercise can slow down the aging process. According to medical experts, at least half of the losses in bodily function that occur between the ages of thirty and seventy can be attributed to lack of exercise—losses such as muscle strength, overall muscle mass, joint mobility, and mineral content in bones (leading to weak, brittle bones). Without exercise, the condition of your body weakens over time, leaving you more vulnerable to illness and age-related deterioration. What happens when you do exercise? The physical problems associated with the aging process are slowed, or even stopped.

2. Exercise can relieve depression. Many mental-health experts consider depression one of the most common psychiatric problems among all age groups, but especially among those ages sixty-five and older. Symptoms of depression include sadness, anger, difficulty sleeping, helplessness, and hopelessness. Researchers have found that people suffering from mild to moderate depression can relieve their symptoms by exercising fifteen to thirty minutes at least every other day.

3. Exercise relieves stress. Stress causes a build-up of hormones and other body chemicals, leaving you feeling anxious and unable to cope. Exercise helps dissipate these chemicals. In addition, physical activity leads to the production and release of hormones called endorphins, which give you a natural high. About an hour after exercising, you may feel more relaxed and peaceful.

"If I miss my walk for a few days, I start to feel anxious and short on patience—the little things in life bother me more. My walking program is good for handling stress."

MARGARET

4. Exercise helps prevent heart disease. People who don't exercise are twice as likely to develop heart disease as people who do. If you exercise regularly, you may reduce your risk of having a fatal heart attack by up to 20 percent. If you already have heart disease or have suffered a heart attack, your doctor has probably told you that exercise is one of the best ways to take care of your heart—and yourself.

5. Exercise increases the "good" cholesterol. You've probably heard a lot about cholesterol, a crystalline substance found in your body tissue and in certain foods. HDL (also known as the "good" cholesterol) is the type that lowers your risk of heart disease. Exercise is an effective way to increase your HDL. While raising your level of HDL, exercise also lowers your level of LDL, or "bad" cholesterol.

"Exercise and eating a healthier diet lowered my cholesterol by thirty points. I feel great, and I know I'm healthier since I made these changes in my life."

GARY

6. Exercise may prevent the most common form of diabetes. Researchers at Stanford University and the University of California at Berkeley have shown that physical activity may help prevent adult-onset diabetes, or noninsulin-dependent diabetes mellitus. One of the benefits of exercise is that it helps control weight (and weight gain is a strong precipitator of adult-onset diabetes). Anyone at risk for diabetes—people who are obese or have high blood pressure, for example—should consider a program of regular exercise.

7. Exercise reduces your risk of getting certain forms of cancer. Research shows that regular exercise, even at a low level of intensity, may help prevent cancer of the breast, colon, and female reproductive organs.

8. Exercise helps you sleep better. If you have a hard time falling asleep or if you're a restless sleeper, regular physical activity can help you get a good night's sleep. People who exercise tend to fall asleep faster, sleep more soundly, and wake up feeling refreshed and ready to start the day.

9. Exercise sharpens your thinking. No matter what age you are, exercise can improve your thinking skills. Studies have shown that people who exercise have sharper memories and better concentration than people who don't exercise.

10. Exercise improves your quality of life. Because exercise makes you stronger and sharper, it can help raise your self-esteem. And when you feel good about yourself, your enthusiasm for life increases. Exercise also gives you more energy to do the things you enjoy—at home, on the job, in the community, and with friends. When you exercise on a regular basis, you're taking responsibility for your own health—something no one can do better than you.

"I have exercised regularly for over twenty years. I feel young, and I have lots of energy to keep up with my busy life."

LYNN

*A*mazing Walkers

Vote Early, Vote Often, Vote Yes for Walkin'

Lawton Chiles loved to walk, and it led him all the way to our nation's capital. As an unknown Southern Democrat, Chiles shook hands and kissed babies while trudging more than 1,000 miles up and down the state of Florida in 1970 in his quest to represent Floridians in Washington. They responded in kind—by walking to the voting booths and casting their ballots for "Walkin' Lawton." When the polls closed, Chiles had won both a seat in the U.S. Senate and his place in history.

If You're over Age Fifty

People over fifty can and should exercise. But if you're over fifty, you may believe that your age, health, and lifestyle make it impossible for you to get fit. Have you fallen for one of the following exercise myths?

MYTH: "I'm too old to exercise."

FACT: The stereotype of the aging person is someone who's frail, dependent, or inactive (or all three). Because our culture values youth, attractiveness, and vigor, most Americans view aging with a sense of dread. But it doesn't have to be this way. Experts now believe that people of any age can gain—or regain—strength, agility, and balance through a program of regular exercise. No one is too old to get in better shape.

Physical activity can prevent, or at least minimize, many of the health problems that might affect you later in life: heart disease, obesity, muscle weakness, or osteoporosis (weakening of bones). In fact, many of these health problems are the result of a sedentary lifestyle—not of "getting old." Regular exercise improves heart and lung fitness, controls weight, and increases muscle strength.

"I have been a good exerciser throughout my life. When I had complications from minor surgery, the doctor was able to treat my condition with less invasive measures than normal. She said that my body—inside and out—seemed younger than my real age. I attribute that to all of my regular exercise."

DIANE

MYTH: "You can't exercise when you're ill."

FACT: If you have a chronic illness or a debilitating disease, you may believe you're too sick to exercise. The good news is you're not! If you have arthritis, osteoporosis, diabetes, or another physical disorder, exercise can help you maintain or improve your muscle strength and your heart and lung fitness. Talk to your doctor about physical activities that are safe and meet your needs.

"When I exercise, my blood sugar stays at a good level and I feel much better."

MARIE

The fact is, aging doesn't automatically mean losing your ability to live your life to the fullest. If you feel tired, weak, or out of shape, don't assume this is a natural and unalterable part of the aging process. The real culprit may be neglect. Have you stopped exercising in favor of spending most of your time sitting? Do you go to bed early and sleep late? Do you watch a lot of TV, spend hours in the car, or sit in front of a computer most of the day?

When you fail to use your muscles, bones, joints, tendons, ligaments, and cartilage, your body begins to waste away. Years of this type of neglect can make you feel sluggish or worn out, and when you feel this way, you tend to rest more, further decreasing your activity and fitness level. In other words, the less you *try* to do, the less you're *able* to do.

You can reverse this trend by becoming active again—it's never too late. In fact, gerontologist Maria Fiatarone, M.D. of Tufts University in Boston proved this point in a study of women over the age of ninety. The elderly women, all of whom were frail and lived in a nursing home, took part in a twelve-week, well-instructed weight-lifting program. The results were dramatic: All of the women greatly increased their strength, including a 200 percent increase in knee flexor strength. Exercise made this possible!

Not only does physical activity increase your strength, it also improves your reaction time (the length of time it takes for you to react mentally and physically to a stimulus). Aging decreases your reaction time, leading to slowed thoughts and movements. Does this matter? Yes, especially if you still drive. Regular exercise helps you retain the quick responses needed whenever you get behind the wheel of a car.

What does all this add up to? Regular exercise is one of the best ways to stay healthy and fit for a lifetime. When you're active, you feel more youthful and have more energy for work and play. There's an old saying that still holds true today: "Exercise adds life to your years . . . and years to your life."

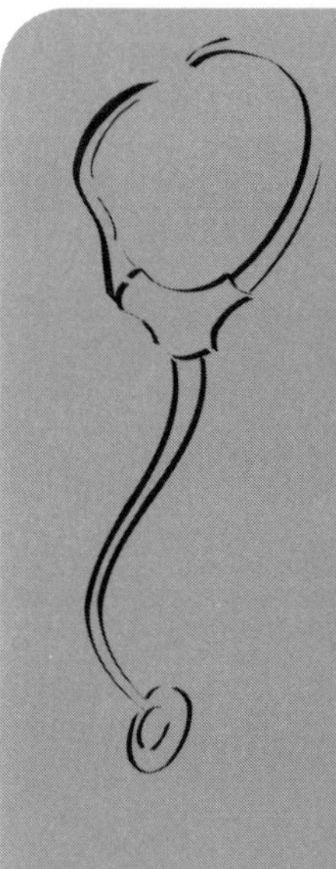

Before starting an exercise program, see your doctor. He or she can help measure your fitness level and design a program that's right for you. This is especially important if you have one or more of the following conditions: high blood pressure, heart trouble, frequent dizzy spells, arthritis, a family history of stroke or heart attack, or a known or suspected disease.

The Activity Pyramid

Take a moment to think about your level of physical activity. Would you characterize it as:

1. **inactive** (haven't thought about activity in years),
2. **sporadic** (active in the summer but not in the winter), or
3. **consistent** (active most of the time, or at least four days a week)?

No matter which category you think you fit into, you can use the Physical Activity Pyramid as a guide for finding creative ways to be active. Developed by the Institute for Research and Education HealthSystem Minnesota, the pyramid is designed to help people understand the importance of a *varied* exercise routine.

If you look at the pyramid on page 19, you'll see that each level represents different types of activities. This is because health experts believe a balanced fitness routine incorporates both aerobic exercise and strength training. What's the difference between them? *Aerobic* exercises use continuous, rhythmic movements, making your heart work harder to deliver oxygen-rich blood to your working muscles. Examples include brisk walking, biking, jogging, or swimming. *Strength training,* on the other hand, involves improving specific muscle groups (abdominals, biceps, and so forth). Lifting hand-held weights or doing push-ups or sit-ups are examples of strength-training exercises.

Some exercises (like yoga and stretching) are designed to improve your *flexibility,* or the ability of your joints and muscles to move through their full range of motion. A well-rounded physical-activity plan includes not only aerobic exercise and strength training but also activities designed to increase your overall flexibility.

Experts also recommend increasing your everyday movement by doing things like taking a walk, getting outdoors, or working in the garden. This means cutting down on sedentary activities like watching TV or sitting for more than thirty minutes at a time.

Each week, try to increase your physical activity using the pyramid as a guide. Here's an explanation of how the four-level pyramid works:

LEVEL 1: This level is made up of everyday activities you should do as often as possible (see page 21 for examples). These movements add extra steps to your day.

LEVEL 2: This level includes both aerobic and recreational exercises, which improve your cardiovascular fitness and your endurance. You could try swimming laps at an indoor pool, for example, or take a tennis class. It's recommended that you do activities from this level three to five times per week.

LEVEL 3: This level consists of leisure activities and exercises designed to improve your strength and flexibility. You might play a round of golf or rent a strength-training video. The goal is to do these types of activities two to three times per week.

LEVEL 4: This level features sedentary activities to cut down on. Avoid sitting for more than thirty minutes at a time. If you sit at work, get up and stretch every half hour or so.

You can use the pyramid to get creative about how you stay active. In a typical week you might:

- take the steps instead of the elevator at work each day
- mall walk on three different days (for more on mall walking, see chapter 5, "Ready to Walk the Walk?")
- go bowling
- take a yoga class
- go out dancing Saturday night, instead of staying at home watching TV

The Activity Pyramid

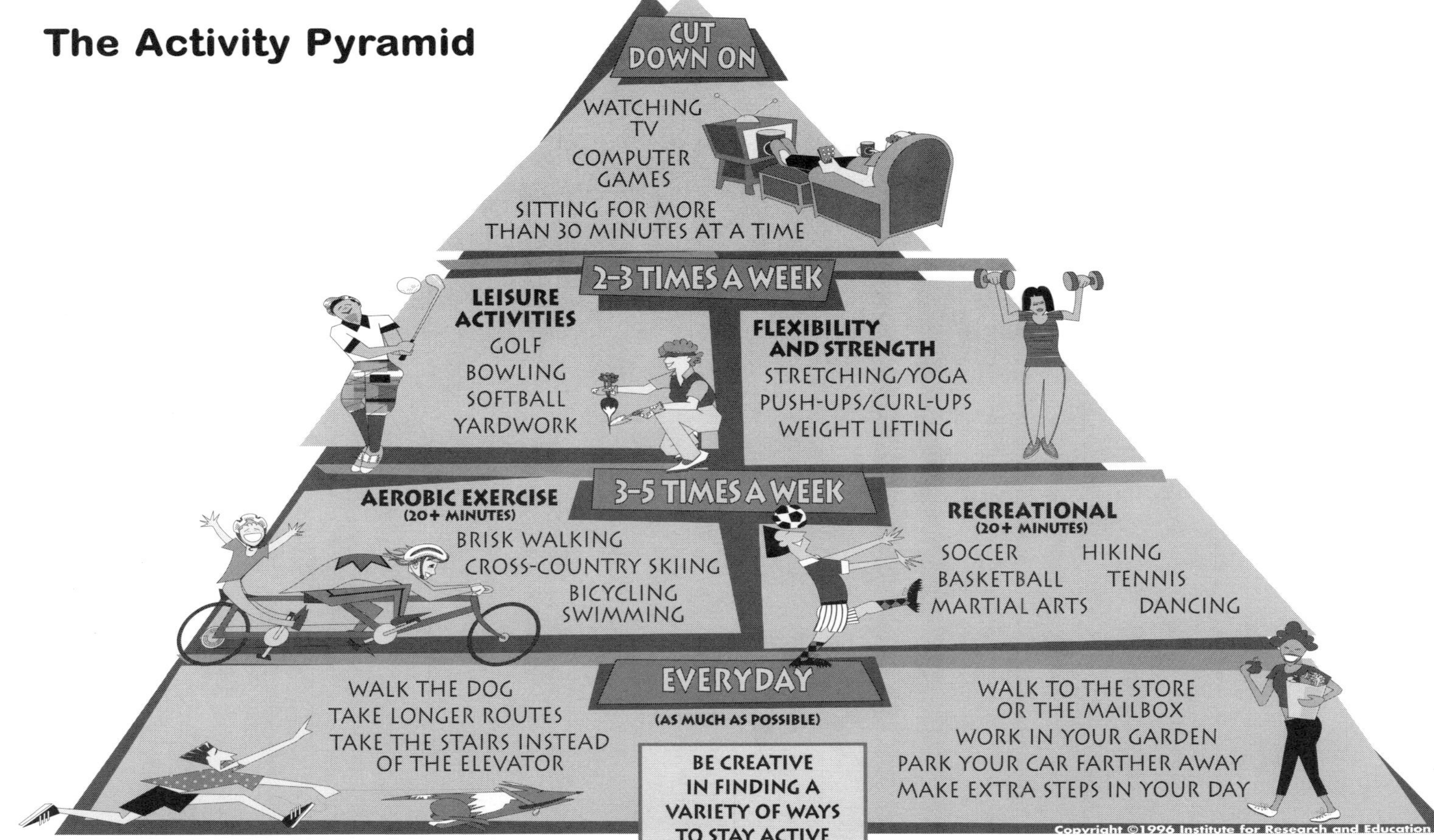

If this sounds like too much, start slow and gradually increase your activity when you feel ready. For example, if you consider yourself inactive, you can begin to get more active by increasing the number of everyday activities found at the base of the pyramid. Try this:

- march in place while talking on the phone
- stretch while standing in line
- walk whenever you can

Start exercising *slowly,* beginning with short periods of ten to fifteen minutes, twice a week. Be sure to listen to your body when you work out. If you feel discomfort or pain, you're trying to do too much too fast. Ease up, take a break, and start again another time. Consult your doctor if you experience chest pain, breathlessness, joint discomfort, or muscle cramps.

Once you're ready, add no more than ten to fifteen minutes of exercise each week. You can eventually increase your workouts to twenty to thirty minutes, three or four times a week, if your doctor says it's okay.

If your physical activity can be characterized as *sporadic,* focus on activities in the *middle* of the pyramid. Make it your goal to become more consistent about exercise. Try this:

- find activities you really enjoy and do them more often
- schedule your exercise sessions by marking the days and times on your calendar or in your day planner (and stick to them)
- set realistic goals for yourself so you have a better chance of reaching them

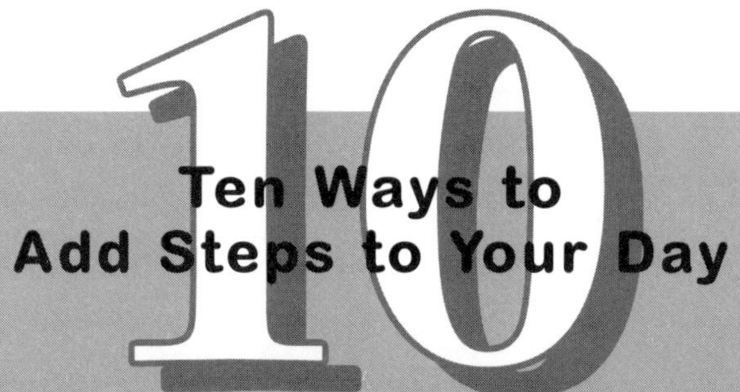

Ten Ways to Add Steps to Your Day

1. Walk instead of drive.
2. Get off the bus a block or two before your stop, then walk.
3. Do housework—make it fun by turning on some music.
4. Go outdoors and play with your children or grandchildren.
5. Bring a pair of walking shoes to work, then take a walk over lunch.
6. Wash the car by hand or sweep out the garage.
7. Mow the lawn (not on a rider mower).
8. Walk up and down the stairs during TV commercials.
9. Hide the remote.
10. Avoid the couch.

If you're *consistent* about exercising, that's great! You can make sure you're getting the most out of your fitness routine by choosing activities from the entire pyramid. Try this:

- include aerobic, strength, and flexibility exercises
- vary your routine to prevent boredom
- explore new activities to maintain your interest in physical fitness

Attention SHOPPERS!

The first suburban shopping center that catered exclusively to shoppers with cars was the Country Club Plaza, built in 1922 in Kansas City, Missouri. Covering 40 acres, with a parking lot designed for 5,500 vehicles, the center's 150 stores and 2,000-seat auditorium were the talk of the town.

If You're over Age Sixty

Park Nicollet HealthSource, in Minnesota, has developed an activity pyramid for people over sixty (see page 25). As you age, your needs and lifestyle may change, but it's still important to stay active. It's up to you to decide which activity pyramid works best for you (talk to your doctor if you have questions or concerns).

Here's how the over-sixty pyramid works:

LEVEL 1: This level is made up of activities that keep you moving throughout the day. Every day you can:

- walk with a friend, grandchild, or dog (if you don't have a dog, become a volunteer dog walker at your local humane society)
- garden, work in the yard, sweep the driveway, or shovel snow
- stay busy by doing leisure activities like bowling or golfing

LEVEL 2: This level features exercises to do throughout the week, including aerobic activities (three to five times per week), balance and flexibility training (three or more times per week), and muscle strengthening (three times per week). Throughout the week you can:

- walk or do water exercises to strengthen your heart and lungs
- stretch or practice yoga to keep your muscles and joints flexible, and to increase your balance (which helps prevent falls)
- lift small hand-held weights to strengthen your muscles, which helps make your daily activities easier

LEVEL 3: Cut down on the sedentary activities in this level. Avoid sitting for more than thirty minutes at a time by taking breaks, getting up and moving around, and stretching as often as possible. You can take frequent breaks when:

- watching TV or renting movies
- sitting in front of the computer for long periods
- doing needlework and crafts

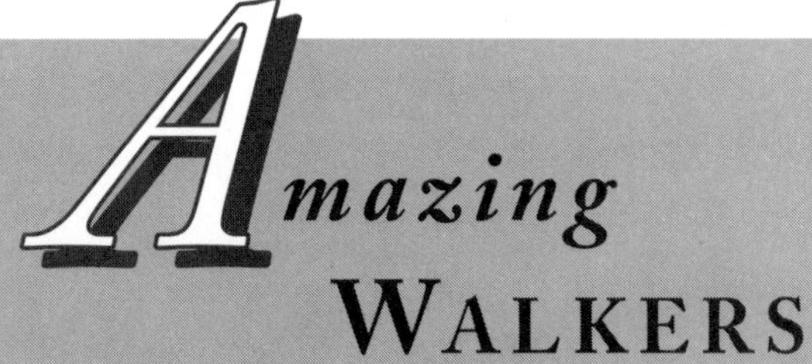

Pioneering Walker

American pioneer "Johnny Appleseed" envisioned apple blossoms fragrantly scenting the air in the New World (America). So from 1797 until his death nearly 50 years later, he walked alone throughout Ohio and Indiana, planting apple orchards. This gentle character, with his tin-pan hat and coffee-sack shirt, left a legacy of folk tales and a lesson for all of us to follow our dreams.

The Activity Pyramid for People over 60

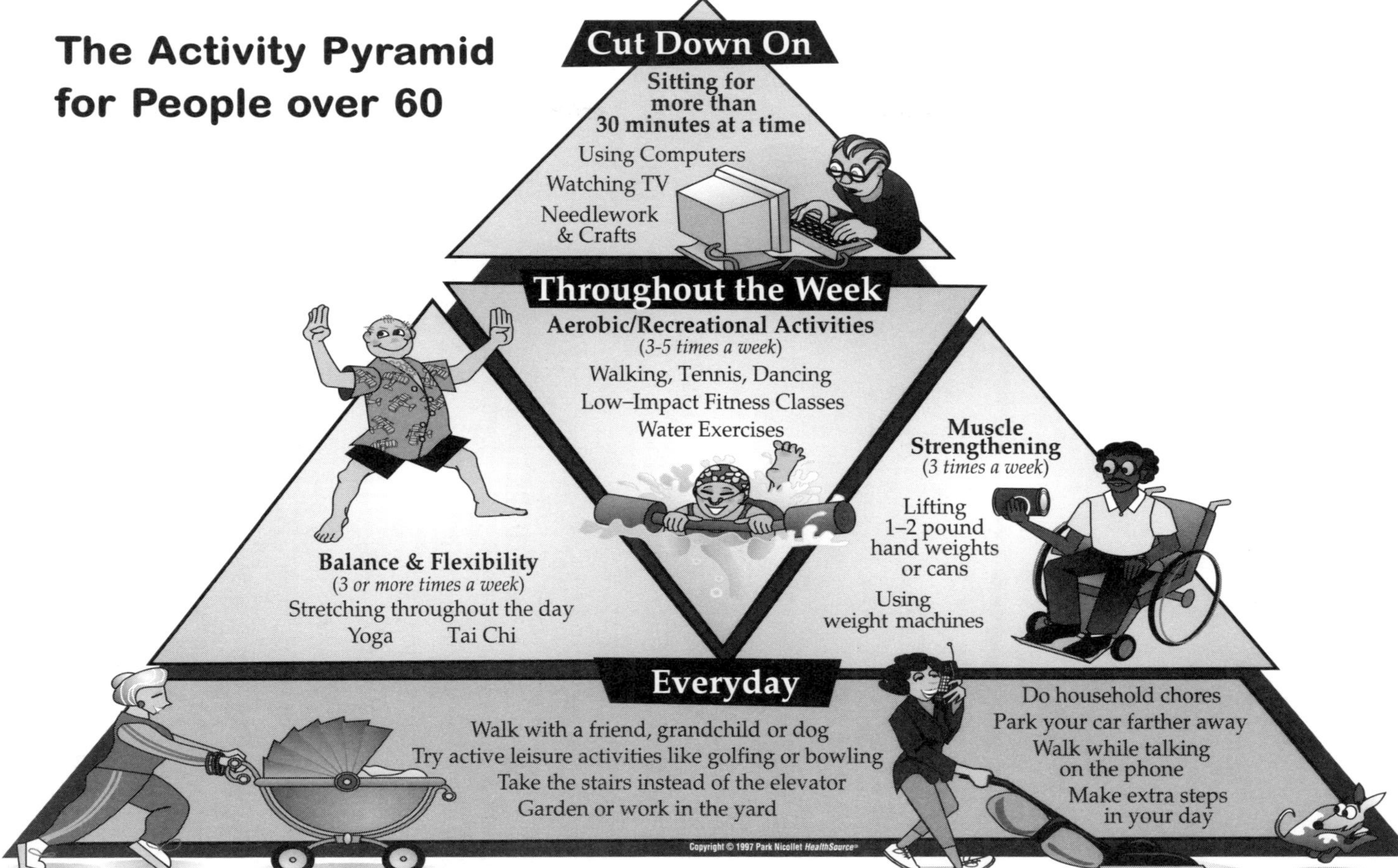

The activities in both pyramids are only suggestions to get you started. Feel free to design a fitness program that suits you and fits your age and needs. If in doubt, consult your doctor or a local fitness expert about ways to increase your level of physical activity.

Above all, have fun when you exercise. A physical fitness routine that feels like a chore is one that won't last. Find activities you look forward to and are motivated to do.

Studies have shown that making a written promise to yourself is a helpful way to get serious about your commitment to exercise. On the following page is a Personal Exercise Contract you can copy, fill out, and sign. Find a witness who not only will watch you sign your contract but also keep in touch with you as you explore fitness activities that are right for you. Ask your witness to check in with you every so often (or, if possible, to exercise with you) and offer encouragement when you need it. Your signed contract can serve as a personal reminder that you care enough about yourself to take steps to improve your health.

"Since I've retired, it's easier to fit my walk in. My advice to younger people is to plan exercise into your day just as you would a meal or brushing your teeth. Even a little is better than nothing."

GERRY

Personal Exercise Contract

I promise to:

1. Exercise at least three times each week.
2. Keep a journal of how I feel during my fitness program.
3. Find an additional physical activity I enjoy.
4. Remain dedicated to improving my health.
5. Reward myself for a job well done.

Signed ________________________________

Witness ________________________________

Date ________________________________

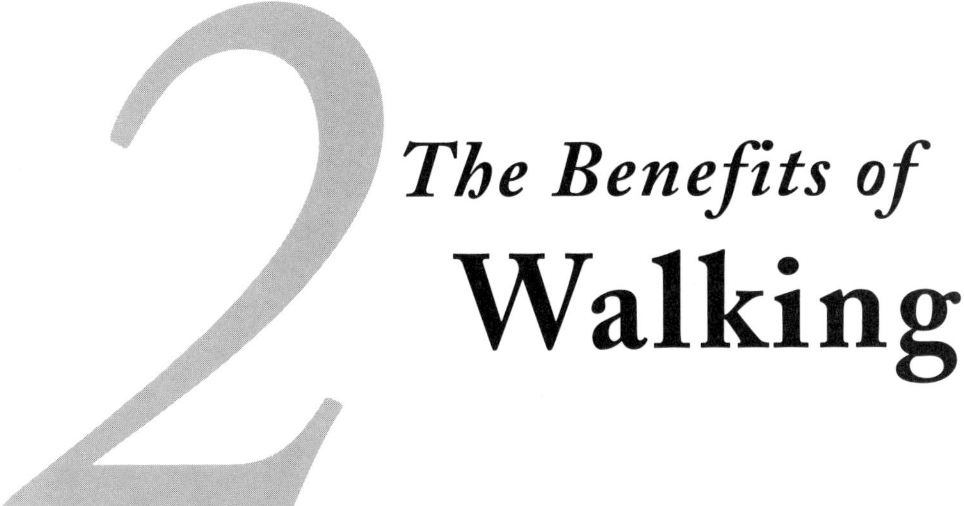

2 The Benefits of Walking

"Walking, not just strolling, is the simplest and also one of the best exercises."
AMERICAN HEART ASSOCIATION

All those walkers out there are onto something. They've figured out that walking is:

1. Easy. You don't have to take lessons to learn how to walk.

2. Fun. It's especially enjoyable with a mall-walking group, family, friends, or your dog.

3. Inexpensive. Few forms of exercise are as simple and affordable. You don't have to invest in a lot of special gear or pay enormous fees at a health club.

4. Beneficial. Walking is a great way to:

- get some aerobic exercise
- improve your mood, mental function, and self-esteem
- lose weight and keep it off
- slow down osteoporosis, or weakening of bones
- relieve stress or feelings of depression

But now there's another good reason to walk: Research suggests that a brisk walk each day can keep older people living longer. In fact, studies of people in their sixties, seventies, and eighties have proven that walking two miles a day cut their mortality rates in half.

"I'm in my sixties now, and I've been walking for years. Each day, I walk to clear my head and tone my body. Walking doesn't hurt me like some other forms of exercise do. If I don't get my walk in, I'm just no fun to be around—that's how much I need it. People say I look younger than my actual age. I think walking has a lot to do with that. I can do this kind of exercise for years to come."

BEVERLY

Benefits by the Mile

So, walking is good for you . . . but is it as good as running, cycling, swimming, rowing, and other kinds of exercise? Yes! Walking is the safest, most practical, and most sensible centerpiece for a fitness program. It clears the mind and reduces stress. A daily fitness walk provides a break from work or boredom and allows you to think, plan, and focus. The mental and physical benefits of walking can be felt within just a few weeks.

Another benefit of walking is that it's a low-impact, low-stress fitness activity. Unlike jogging, it doesn't produce a lot of wear-and-tear on your knees. Walking puts less stress on your muscles, joints, ligaments, and bones than many other forms of exercise, lowering your risk of injury.

Walking regularly conditions your heart, improves overall circulation, augments lung capacity, reduces blood pressure, and burns calories effectively. If you have high blood pressure or are obese, you probably realize these conditions are high risk factors for both stroke and heart attack. Walking helps lower blood pressure and weight, decreasing your risk.

Walking improves muscle strength, too. Because walking uses most of the major muscle groups, it helps firm your buttocks and trim your thighs. The rhythmic arm swing that naturally accompanies walking helps to work your chest, shoulder, and arm muscles. Proper walking in good posture also strengthens abdominal and back muscles. The end result? You feel and look stronger, fitter, and more toned.

"I feel better when I exercise, and I think it becomes more important the older you get. Some days when I'm dragging, I take a brisk walk to renew my energy. I feel so good afterward!"

JUDY

Walking and Weight Loss

In America today, one in every three people is overweight. Why? Most experts say one of the main factors is inactivity. The truth is, overweight people in our society tend to be less physically active than people of average body weight. Lack of exercise can lead to weight gain, and weight gain can lead to lack of exercise (it's harder to work out or do daily activities when you're carrying extra weight around). The cycle of inactivity and weight gain becomes a vicious circle.

Walking not only builds muscle but also *burns calories.* Studies have shown that walking burns almost as many calories as jogging, and since you probably can walk for a longer period than you can jog, walking may help you burn more calories during each exercise session. If you walk for thirty minutes at a moderate pace, you can burn anywhere from 90 to 120 calories. You build your muscles and reduce the size of your fat-storing cells—this helps you slim down. So say good-bye to your love handles—walking takes the weight off!

"My doctor told me to take a walk . . . and he meant vigorously. I now walk (at the mall) for my health. I go for one hour every day, and I've lost twenty-five pounds in nine months."

LES

Amazing Walkers

Walking on Air

Does that old pull of gravity weigh you down? Not so for Cosmonaut Aleksei Leonov, who became the first human to walk in space. Leonov stepped out of his *Voskhodz* spacecraft on March 18, 1965, and strode quickly into the history books.

Just a few months later on June 3, American astronaut Major Edward Higgins White II opened the hatch of *Gemini 4* and strolled into space. At 120 miles above the earth, he walked in space for 20 minutes, attached to his spacecraft by a 25-foot cord.

But these two walking achievements pale in comparison to Neil Alden Armstrong's momentous moonwalk. Armstrong and Lt. Colonel Edwin E. "Buzz" Aldrin, Jr. lifted off from Kennedy Space Center in Cape Canaveral, Florida, on *Apollo 11* in 1969. On July 20, they landed on the moon's *Sea of Tranquility* in the lunar module *Eagle.* Armstrong descended the ladder to the moon's surface, uttering the now epic phrase, "That's one small step for man, one giant leap for mankind."

Walking and Your Heart

Because brisk walking is a form of aerobic exercise, it helps strengthen your heart muscle (at any age). Every year, millions of Americans suffer heart attacks, and unfortunately about half of them don't survive. Regular exercise plays a significant role in lowering your risk of having a fatal heart attack.

Those who survive a heart attack are usually encouraged to begin a cardiac rehabilitation program that includes quitting smoking, eating a low-fat diet, and making exercise a part of their life. Walking is an important component of most cardiac rehabilitation programs. This form of exercise is generally considered safe for cardiac patients, as long as their progress is monitored by a doctor.

"I was sixty-seven when I had my heart attack. I had triple bypass surgery right away. The doctors told me I'd have to quit smoking, eat right, and get in shape. They also told me about the mall-walking program in my town. Now I go a few times each week. What surprised me was how easy it was to start feeling fit again. I have more energy than ever. I see the same people at the mall all the time. I wave or say hi. I see young people there, too. We encourage each other."

BILL

Walking and Arthritis

If you have arthritis, you may be hesitant to walk because it might cause you pain. Keep in mind that, in many cases, people with arthritis *should* exercise. The increased physical activity can play an important role in decreasing the severity of the arthritis. Talk to your doctor about starting a walking program: Moving your joints may be the best way to heal them.

> *"My doctor advised me not to run, jump, or lift weights above my shoulders—it's too hard on my joints. He said that walking was the best exercise for me."*
>
> *JILL*

Today's arthritis doctors appreciate the need for exercise—regardless of the type of arthritis or its extent. They realize many of the signs and symptoms of arthritis in and around the joints are a consequence of failure to keep the joint moving to at least some degree. Ligaments and tendons lose tensile strength very gradually, capsules of joints become loose, and cartilage tends to wear. All these are a consequence of what can be called "stress deprivation" or "exercise deficiency": failure to achieve mechanical stimulation of all joint structures throughout the body. Of course, pain often restricts movement, but exercising up to whatever the limits are, under the guidance of a good doctor, can relieve and improve almost any patient with arthritis.

Walking and the Activity Pyramids

The wonderful thing about walking is that it can fit into every level of the activity pyramids (for more about the pyramids, see chapter 1, "Why Is Exercise Important?"). Take the pyramid on page 19 as an example: Level 1 is all about walking—as a way to add steps to your day. Level 2, which focuses on aerobic exercise, offers brisk walking as an exercise option. And Level 3 includes leisure activities like golf, which involves a fair amount of walking, unless you use a golf cart. Once you start walking for fitness, you'll find that your daily activities are less strenuous and easier to accomplish—this means you'll be less inclined to sit for long periods (a Level 4 "activity" to cut down on).

The activity pyramids encourage you to do some type of physical activity every day, and walking is one form of exercise that's easy to do on a regular basis. Because walking is so enjoyable, you may find that daily exercise is more rewarding and pleasurable than you ever thought possible.

No pain, no gain . . . don't believe it for a minute! It's a myth that you have to exercise to the point of pain to achieve beneficial effects. Exercise consistently, rather than focusing on short-term intensity. And don't think walking isn't intense enough to make you fit. Walking truly is an excellent form of exercise; it's a sound and sane option in a fitness-crazed world.

DID YOU KNOW . . .

How you carry yourself plays a big role in building and maintaining your self-confidence. And how you walk influences the way you think and feel.

Get into the habit of carrying yourself with confidence and walking with authority. How? Hold your head high, with your chin up and eyes forward and focused; your shoulders should be drawn back from your chest. Swing your arms and walk with a bounce in your step. Avoid slouching and dragging your feet. Soon you'll feel more positive, upbeat, and energetic. Your self-confidence—the most important mental ingredient for success—will soar.

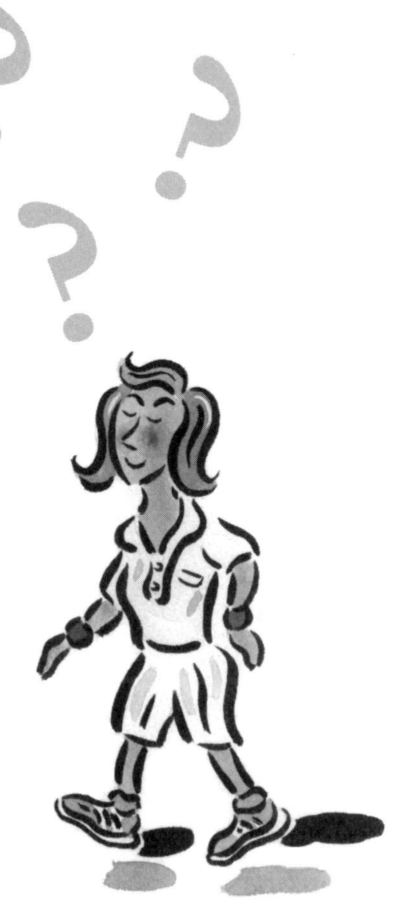

3 *Flexibility and Stretching:* Loosen Up!

"The body is shaped, disciplined, honored, and in time, trusted."
MARTHA GRAHAM

A well-rounded physical activity plan includes exercises that increase your flexibility, and walking (while beneficial) isn't one of these exercises. What to do? Start stretching. Stretching increases your flexibility from head to toe.

When your body is flexible, your muscles and tendons are more pliable, and this allows your joints to move through their full range of motion. One benefit of flexibility is a better body shape—you'll improve your body symmetry and posture, and you might even start to look leaner. Another benefit is that stretching helps your muscles relax. This is especially important for regular walkers because walking causes the muscles at the back of the legs to contract, and repeated contractions can shorten these muscles. The result is that your calves, for example, may become too tight, which increases your risk of an exercise injury. To avoid this, keep your muscles strong, supple, and pliable through regular stretching.

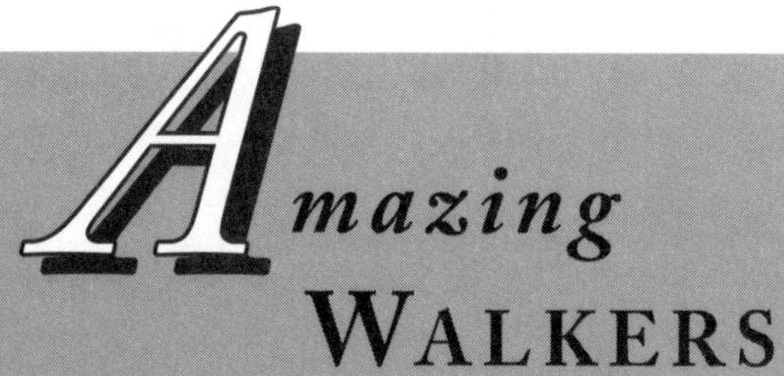

Watch Your Step

No one wants to stumble and fall, but when you're walking a tightrope, there's simply no room for error. Madame Adolphe of Paris, the world's first female tightrope walker, knew this when she wowed the crowds in New York City in 1819 with her walking prowess. More than a century later, New Yorkers would be awed by the French again, when Philippe Petit walked between two towers of the World Trade Center in 1974 at a heart-stopping height of 1,350 feet.

More Good Reasons to Stretch

When you mall walk or do any other type of physical activity, do you always stretch beforehand? You should!

Think of your body as a car that has sat out in the cold all night: Before you can zip off to the mall, you need to give the vehicle some time to warm up so it can perform better. Stretching is a warm-up for your muscles: It helps prepare them for the strenuous activity you're about to do. Following are some more benefits of stretching.

1. **It improves your circulation.** Stretching brings more oxygen and nutrients to your muscles.

2. **It helps prevent injuries.** A stretched muscle resists stress better than an unstretched muscle.

3. **It increases your range of motion.** You'll be able to reach farther or higher.

4. **It reduces muscle tension and pain.** You'll feel more relaxed.

5. **It improves coordination.** Your movements will be freer and easier.

6. **It allows for better sports performance.** Whether you walk, bike, swim, or do any other physical activity, regular stretching can help your body work more efficiently.

7. **It improves your body awareness.** Once you begin to work certain muscle groups, you'll have a better sense of their strength and their limitations.

Flexibility can be improved at any age with appropriate training, although not everyone will improve at the same rate. Just remember to take it slow and don't expect instant results.

"I know I need to stretch more than I do. It gets me ready to exercise and more flexible for my other daily activities."

MIKE

The good news about stretching is you don't have to be in top physical condition or have great athletic skill to do it. Stretching can be done almost anywhere and at any time, even in bed. (Sleeping under an electric blanket or down comforter warms your whole body, an ideal prelude for in-bed stretching exercises.) You can stretch at work, in your car, and while waiting for the bus or walking down the street.

"I just trained through an injury.
Stretching helps prevent injuries and
warms up my muscles before exercise."

DALE

Amazing Walkers

Record Setters

Edward Payson Weston had a dream. He wanted to be the first person to walk across the United States, coast to coast. Starting off from New York City in March of 1909, he reached San Francisco 104 days and 3,795 miles later. Seventy years old at the time of his transcontinental walking adventure, Weston made the return trip one year later, walking from Los Angeles to New York City in 76 days—beating his own record.

Maurizio Damilano of Italy also had a dream. How far could he walk in an hour? In two hours? Farther than anyone else? In October of 1992, he walked a world-record 18 miles, 660 yards in two hours.

How to Stretch

When done correctly, stretching feels good. You shouldn't challenge yourself to see how far you can stretch. It's not necessary to try to increase the degree of stretching each day. The key to proper stretching is regularity and relaxation.

Never do your stretch routine "cold." You've seen commercials about engine wear in cars: The same thing happens in your body. When muscles, tendons, and ligaments haven't been active for a time, they're stiff and more resistant to stretching. Joints that haven't been stretched don't have as much lubricating fluid between the surfaces of bone and cartilage, and are much more prone to injury. Before you start stretching, walk around for a bit to get yourself moving (or just march in place). After a few minutes of this, your body will be warmer and ready to stretch.

Stretching is easy to learn, but there's a right way and a wrong way to do it. The right way is a relaxed, sustained stretch *held for at least twenty seconds,* with attention focused on the muscles being stretched. Stretching rapidly, bouncing up and down, or stretching to the point of pain will do more harm than good.

Start your stretching easy—no bouncing. Stretch to a point where you feel mild tension. Then concentrate on relaxing as you hold that point. The feeling of tension should subside as you hold the position, so you can slightly increase the degree of the stretch. If the tension doesn't subside, ease off slightly and find a degree of tension that's comfortable. Correctly done, stretching shouldn't be painful.

After easy stretching, move slowly a fraction of an inch further until you again feel mild tension. Keep the stretch under control. As tension diminishes, continue to increase the stretch gradually.

Don't hold your breath while you stretch. Your breathing should be slow, rhythmic, and controlled. To do a forward-bending stretch, exhale as you bend forward, and breathe slowly as you hold the stretch. If a stretch position inhibits natural breathing, you aren't relaxed. Ease up on the stretch, so you can breathe naturally.

When you stretch muscle fibers too far (by bouncing or over-stretching), a nerve reflex is triggered, sending a signal to the muscles to contract. You have a similar involuntary muscle reaction when you touch something hot—without even having to think about it, your body pulls away from the heat to prevent injury. When you stretch too far, you tighten the very muscles you're trying to stretch.

"I stretch first thing in the morning on most days, and it feels great now. At first, it took my body time to get adjusted to the routine. Stretching makes me feel stronger, and surprisingly taller. I guess it has to do with my posture, which is now better. Even though I'm older, I don't feel like I'm 'shrinking' like some old folks."

GERI

A Stretching Routine

You can perform the following stretching routine at least once a day, ideally before and after you exercise.

Standing with your head and neck in slight extension (i.e., looking at where the ceiling meets the wall), lower your chin to your chest, then roll your head to the right. Stretch as far as you can to the right side, then bring your chin back to your chest. Next, roll your head to the left, then bring your chin to your chest once more. Repeat ten times.

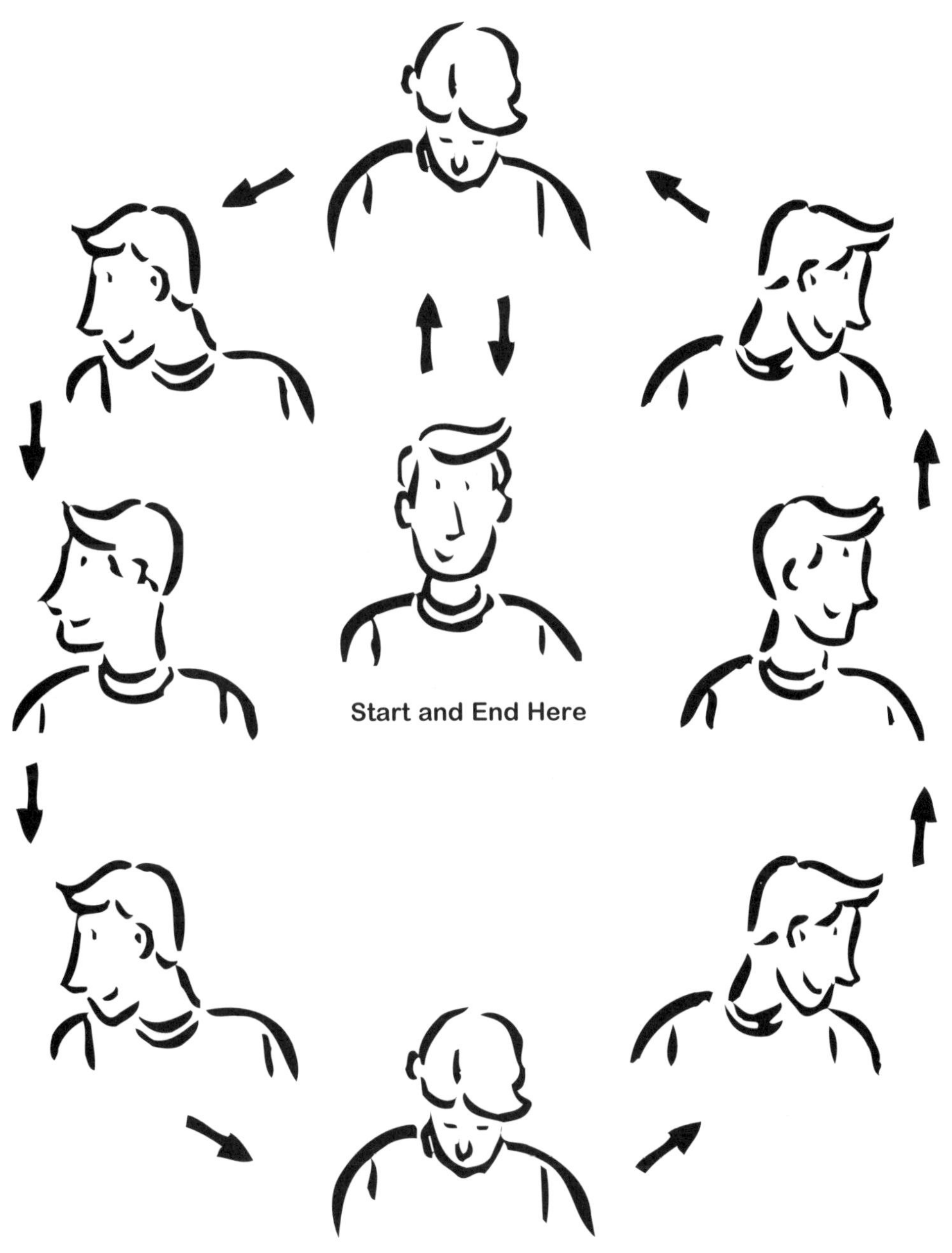
Start and End Here

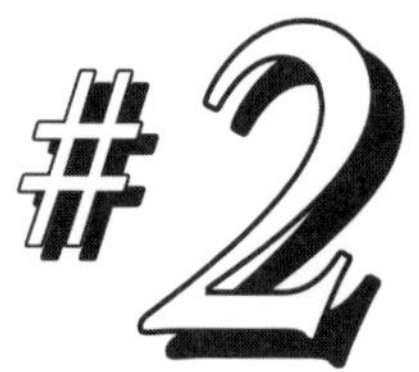

Keeping your right arm straight, slowly raise it above your head, rotating the arm to make as complete and large a circle as possible in a vertical plane. Rotate your arm one revolution over twenty seconds. Repeat and then do the opposite arm. Alternatively, both arms can be stretched at once.

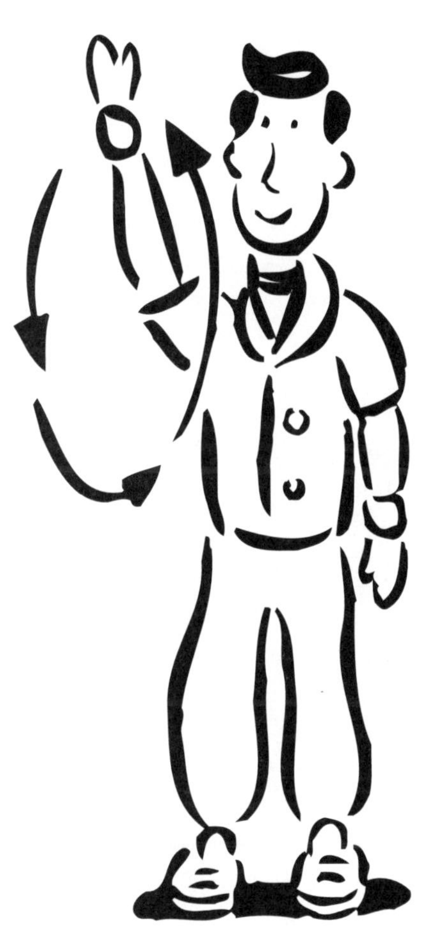

Flex your neck to the side, bringing your ear as close to your shoulder as you can without lifting your shoulder. Then flex your whole spine to the side, reaching with your hand as far down the side of that leg as is comfortable. Hold twenty seconds. Repeat on the left side.

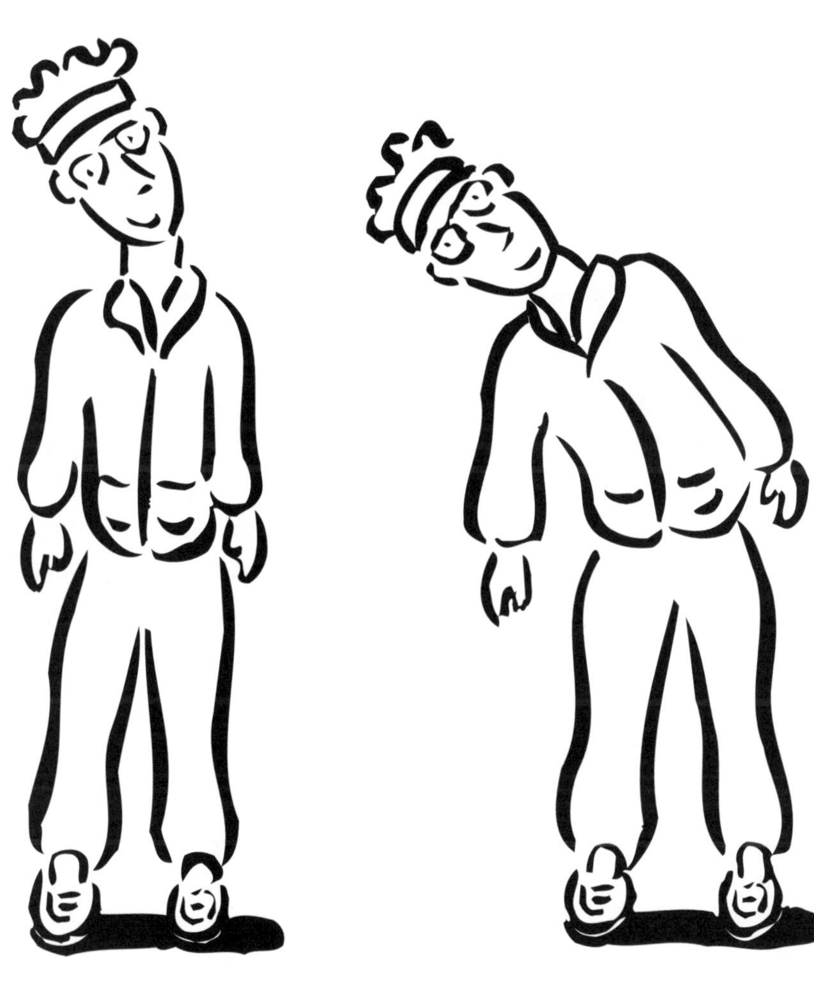

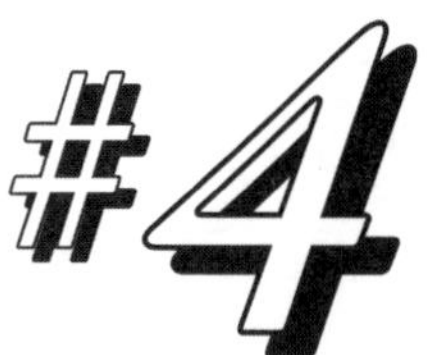

While standing with your feet spaced one foot apart, rotate your head as far as possible to the right, keeping your shoulders square over your hips. After a few seconds, turn your shoulders and rotate your whole spine, looking as far as you can behind you to your right. Hold for twenty seconds. Repeat in the opposite direction.

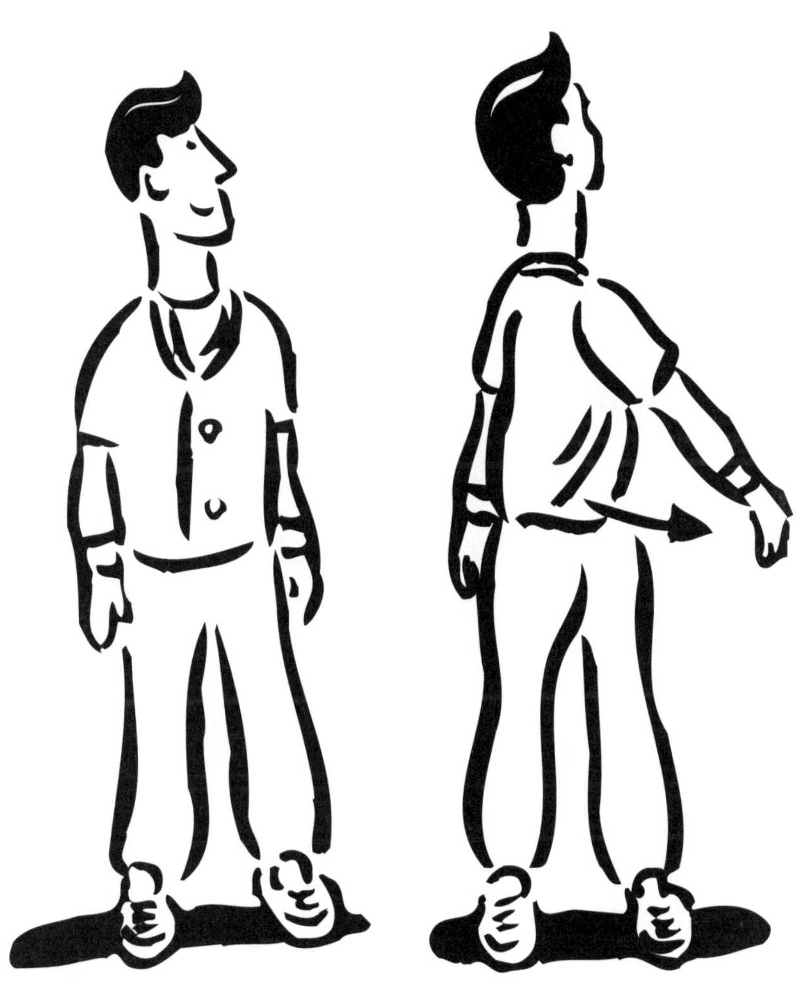

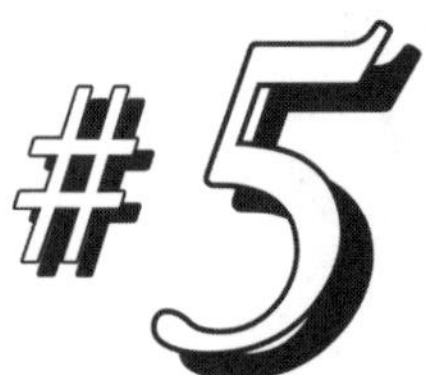

Put your right hand up near your right shoulder. With your left hand and arm, push the right elbow upward, pointing it toward the ceiling. Keep your right arm relaxed in a passive stretch, letting the left hand cause the stretch. Hold for twenty seconds. Repeat for the left elbow, using the right arm to assist.

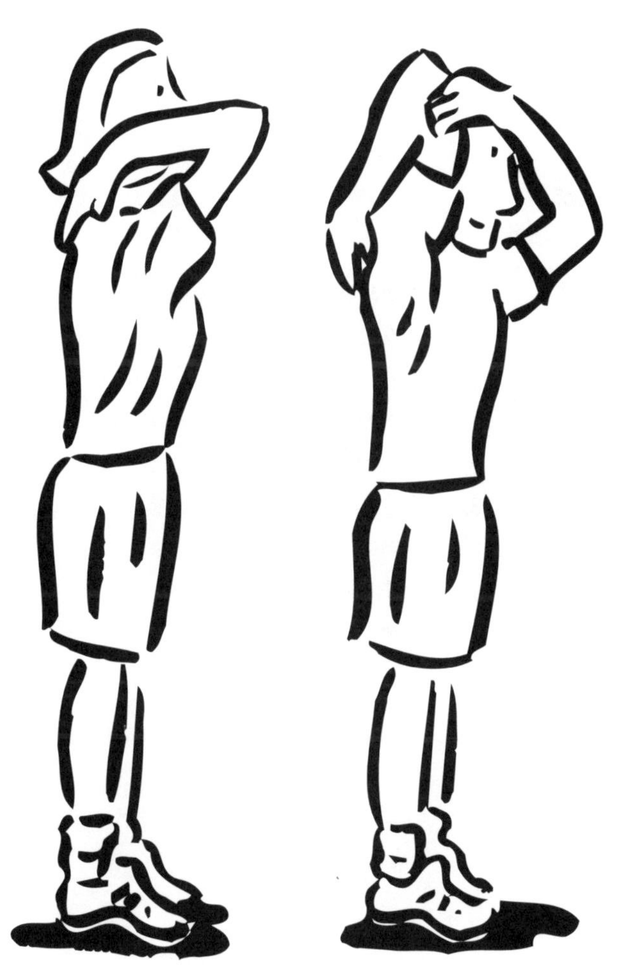

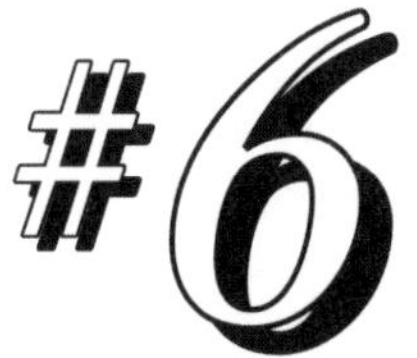

Standing erect with your right arm at your side, reach behind your back with your left hand and grasp your right wrist. Lift your right forearm as parallel to the floor as possible behind your back. Hold for twenty seconds. Repeat on the opposite side.

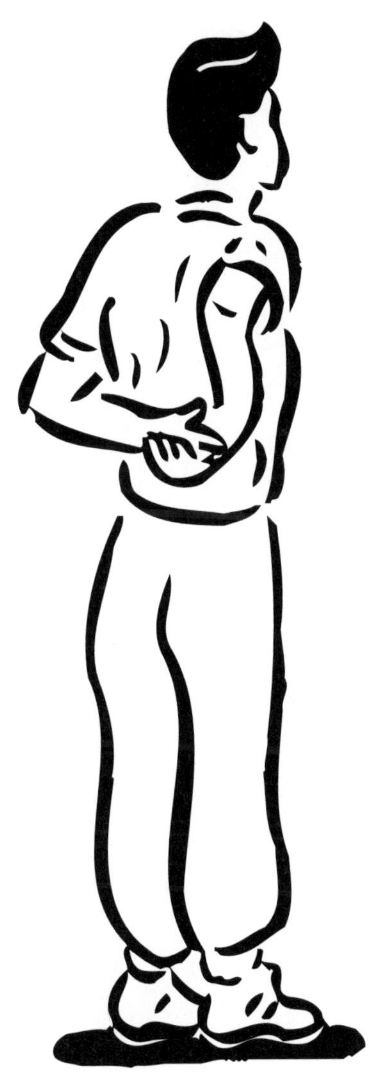

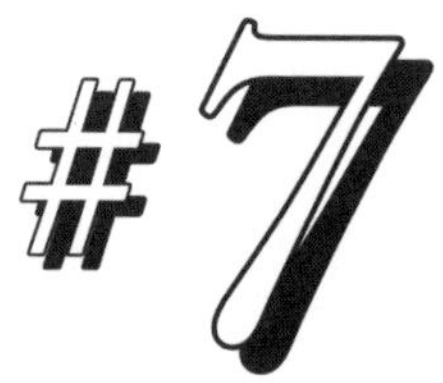

Standing beside a table, kitchen counter, or chair, lift one leg and rest your heel on the surface. Keeping your leg straight, lean forward, reaching for your toes on that foot. Gently pull your toes toward you. Hold for twenty seconds. Repeat on the opposite side.

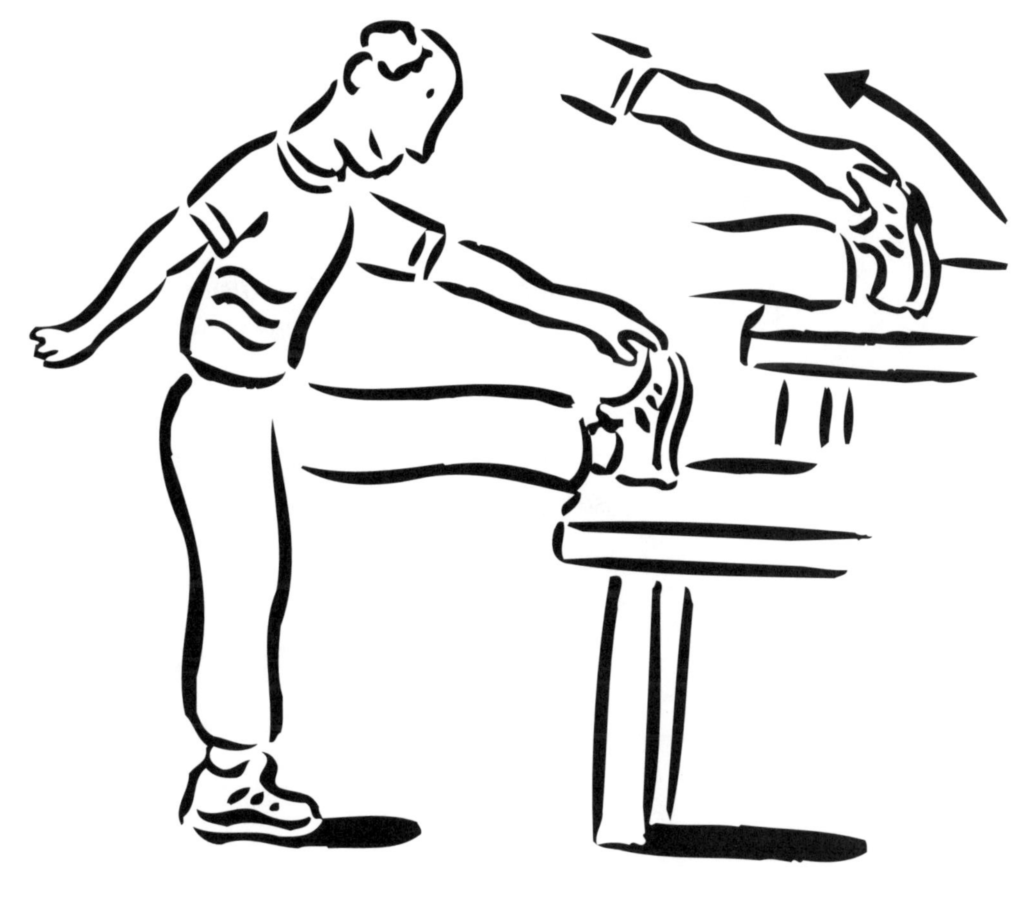

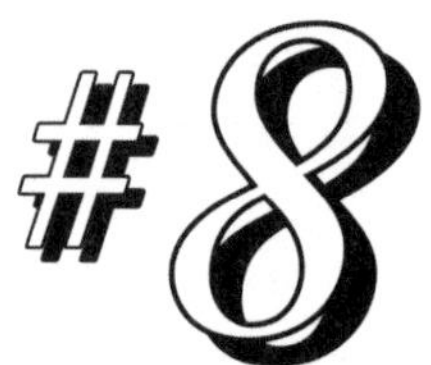

Standing on your left foot (using a wall or post if necessary for balance), grasp your right foot at the toes or ankle. Bring your heel up to your buttock until you feel gentle tension in your right thigh. Hold twenty seconds. Repeat on the opposite side.

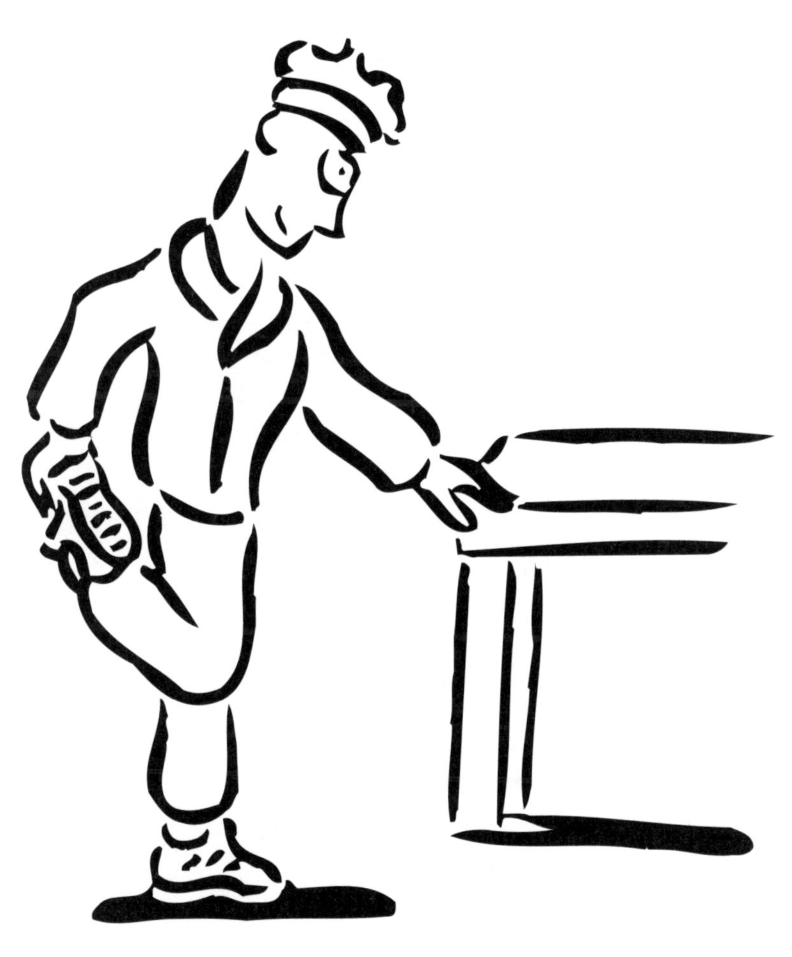

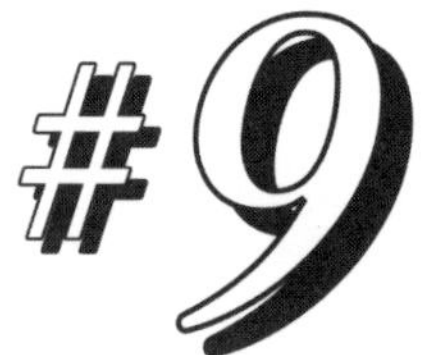

Standing on your left foot, grasp the toes of your right foot with your left hand. Using your right hand as necessary, lift your knee up and out as far as is comfortable. Your hip should be extended laterally. Stand as erect as possible for twenty seconds. Repeat on the opposite side. (If you experience knee pain, do not do this stretch.)

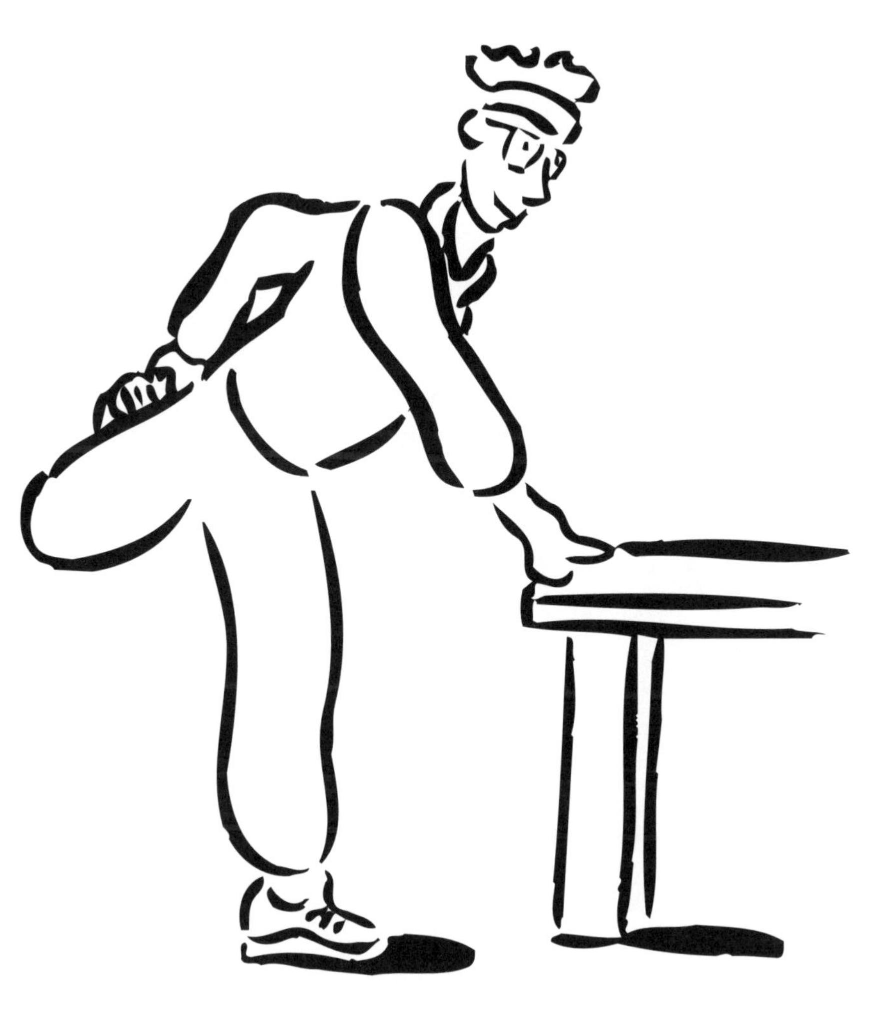

#10

Place both hands on a countertop or other stable surface. Put your right leg in front of your left, bending your right knee. Lean forward on your right leg, using the counter for support, and stretch the back of your left calf as much as possible. Hold twenty seconds. Switch legs and repeat.

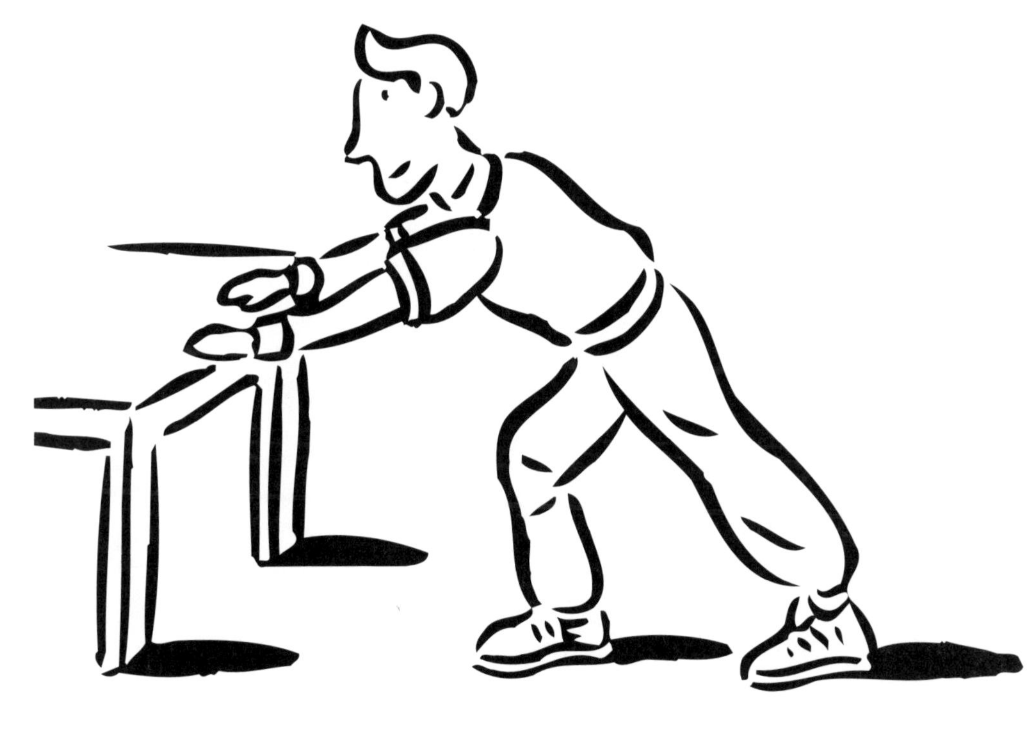

#11

Spread your legs apart, then reach for the floor. Hold for twenty seconds, stretching the inside of both thighs.

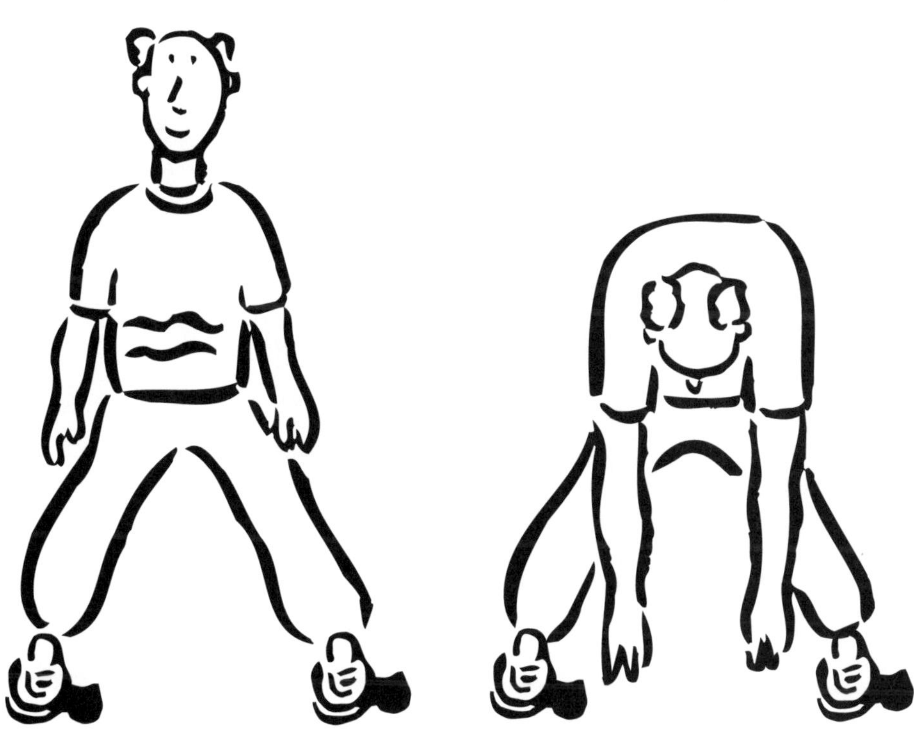

4 On-the-Go Gear

"A good pair of shoes is the only 'special equipment' required by the walker."

THE PRESIDENT'S COUNCIL ON PHYSICAL FITNESS AND SPORTS

You're thinking about taking a walk, so you grab the old running shoes you haven't worn in ten years and you're set to go . . . right? Wrong! People in the walking community have learned that wearing the *right* shoes—not just any old shoes—enhances a walker's comfort and performance.

There's truth to the saying: "You wouldn't wear basketball shoes to run, so why would you wear running shoes to walk?" This goes for court shoes, aerobic shoes, and everyday shoes as well. If you're going to walk, invest in a good pair of walking shoes. Your feet will thank you!

Your Walking Shoes

If you need to purchase walking shoes, start by visiting an athletic store or shoe store that has a wide selection, and bring along the pair of socks you typically wear while working out. (FYI: Always use cotton socks to absorb perspiration when you exercise. The higher the percentage of cotton the better.)

Make sure to tell the salesperson you specifically need walking shoes, then try on several pairs, with the socks you brought. It's best to find a pair of shoes that allows your feet to "breathe," such as shoes made of nylon mesh.

Once the shoes are laced up, move your toes around to see if you have enough freedom of movement. If your toes rub against any part of the shoes, the pair is not a good fit.

The heels of the shoes should have extra padding to help absorb shock. Look for good arch support, too—the shoes should elevate your heels one-half to three-quarters of an inch above the soles of your feet. Be sure you have enough traction for sudden stops.

At the store, walk on a hard surface like linoleum, not just on carpeting, so you really put the shoes to the test. Are the shoes comfortable? Do they pinch anywhere? Do they give you enough support? Can you afford them?

For added comfort, consider buying extra padding or heel and arch supports. These devices will help aid shock absorption.

"After trying on several brands, I finally chose a good walking shoe. It flexes easily from toe to heel and matches the arch of my foot. I tried the shoes for one month and loved them."

NANCY

Treat your walking shoes with care, so they last. Use these shoes only for walking, not for other forms of exercise, errands, or yard work. After each exercise session, air your shoes outdoors in indirect sunlight with the laces removed. If you want, sprinkle the inside of your shoes with deodorizing powder or baking soda to freshen them.

If your walking shoes get dirty or wet, never throw them in the washer or dryer. Instead, wipe them down with a damp cloth and dry them outdoors. It's also possible to dry them with a hairdryer—just make sure it's on a low setting.

How long will your shoes last? It depends on how often and how hard you exercise in them. Shoes typically lose one-third of their ability to absorb shock for every 500 miles of use. If you wear your shoes for about five hours per week (during stretching, warm-ups, walks, and cool-downs), you'll need to replace them every six months or so.

You'll know your shoes are ready to be retired if the sides are sagging, the heels are worn, or the linings are frayed or torn. If only the insoles are worn down, you can buy new ones at your local drugstore.

No matter how good your shoes are, there may be times when you get a blister or callus. Carry along antibacterial ointment and adhesive bandages, so you can continue walking, if you choose to.

*A*mazing Walkers

Walking for a Cause

Many walkers shared Martin Luther King's dream—and more than 250,000 of them joined the peaceful activist in his 1963 "March on Washington" in support of civil rights legislation. Two years later, another 25,000 walkers marched from Selma to Montgomery, Alabama, as part of a voter registration drive. King's dream galvanized many Americans to get out of their armchairs and walk for freedom.

Workout Wear

When choosing what to wear on your walk, remember that comfort is more important than style. Make sure your outfit allows you to move easily and to stay cool as your body temperature rises.

You may want to dress in layers that you can remove as you warm up during your walk. Start with a base layer of cotton clothing such as leggings and a T-shirt. Add sweatpants and a sweatshirt on top, if you'd like.

"I like to walk in comfortable clothes so I can move easily. Oftentimes I wear two layers, so as I warm up I can take off my sweatshirt."

DON

Women who walk have one clothing requirement: an athletic bra. Athletic bras not only provide support and protect tender breast tissue but also help wick the sweat away from your body. You'll be much more comfortable if you wear one. Look for materials such as lycra, stretch cotton, or spandex.

One advantage to mall walking is that the mall's indoor temperature will remain comfortable and consistent. You won't have the added burden of outerwear such as a rain slicker, a hat, or gloves. And you won't have to bring along sunglasses, sunscreen, or bug spray either.

Another advantage is that many malls provide storage lockers for customers. During winter, you can rent a locker to store your coat, hat, and any other clothing and accessories you don't want to carry. During the work week, you can stop at the mall at the end of the day to do your workout; just bring along your exercise wear and stash your work clothes in a locker. This way, you don't have to go home and change first.

If you enjoy shopping or eating at a restaurant after your walk around the mall, take along extra clothing and store it in a rented locker. (You can also place your purse or wallet here, if the lockers are secure.) You'll be more comfortable if you have clean, dry clothing to change into after a workout. Besides, some restaurants may have a dress code that won't allow shorts or other casual wear.

Walking Accessories

The following optional items help make walking at the mall or anywhere else more enjoyable. They also keep you motivated!

- **A pedometer.** This device records your mileage (it measures the number of steps you take in feet).
- **An ACCUSPLIT Eagle Activity Pedometer.** This newer technological device measures every step you take throughout the day. You can clip it on first thing in the morning to get an accurate count of how many steps you take during the day, with a goal of reaching 10,000 steps before you go to bed (this number indicates you're active). Two models are available: One simply counts your steps, while the other counts your steps, the miles you've walked, and the calories you've burned. For more information about the ACCUSPLIT Eagle Activity Pedometer, call 1-800-935-1996. If you're online, go to *http://www.accusplit.com.*
- **A water bottle.** Drinking water during your workout is a great way to stay hydrated, so you might want to carry a water bottle with you on walks. For more information about the importance of water, see chapter 6, "Staying Cool."
- **A fanny pack.** A small pack like this can hold things you might need on your walk—lip balm, spare change, your driver's license, a credit card, extra socks, antibacterial ointment, adhesive bandages, or aspirin.

- **Hand or ankle weights.** These types of weights help increase the intensity of your workouts, but make sure you're ready to handle them. Talk to your doctor first and start with light weights—you can always add more weight later.
- **Headphones.** Listening to music tapes, CDs, the news, or talk radio can help pass the time as you walk. Plus, this is a great opportunity to focus on what you're listening to—no interruptions! Tip: Your local library is a great resource for tapes and CDs.
- **A walking stick or cane.** These items help seniors or people with disabilities or injuries to balance and feel more stable and secure.

"I like to listen to books on tape while I walk. Typically, I walk for about an hour, then meet with friends to enjoy a cup of coffee. There's no excuse to miss walking at the mall—the 'weather' is always nice."

DAPHNE

DID YOU KNOW . . .

It's a myth that you have to toughen up your feet for walking. Blisters and thick calluses are a sign of problems, not a sign that you're getting in better shape! If you have these problems, check to see if your shoes fit properly and you're taking good care of your feet. Good foot care includes trimming your toenails regularly, washing your feet after walking, and "airing" your feet so your skin has a chance to breathe.

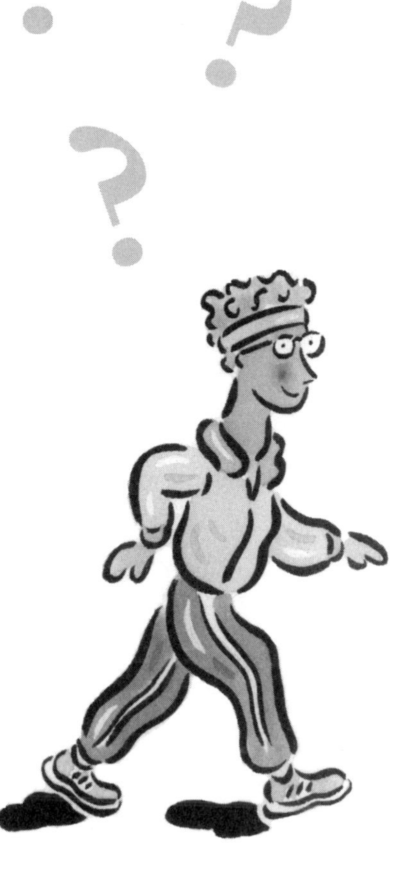

5 Ready to Walk the Walk?

"A journey of a thousand miles begins with a single step."
CHINESE PROVERB

Are you ready to begin your journey? Before you get started, ask yourself what kind of shape you're in. Are you in good shape? Okay shape? Bad shape? Be honest about this. Whether you're in good shape or not-so-good shape, it's best to consult a doctor before starting an exercise program, especially if you've been inactive for a while.

A Program for Beginners

If you're just starting to walk for fitness, don't push yourself too hard, too fast. The first time out, try to walk for about ten minutes. Even at a slow pace you can burn anywhere from sixty to eighty calories. If you want to follow a specific program, you can use the guidelines on page 81. Your goal will be to walk two or three times per week, for a ten-week period. After ten weeks, you should be able to walk briskly nonstop for a full twenty minutes three times per week.

"Walking is so good for you, and I recommend it as something you should do. I wasn't always in good shape—I took my time and started slow. Now, I walk for one hour each day, Monday through Saturday, and have for the last five years. For me, walking gets the juices flowing!"

CATHY

Guidelines for New Walkers

Week 1
Walk briskly* 1 minute.
Walk slowly** 2 minutes.
Repeat 5 times.
Total time: 15 minutes

Week 2
Walk briskly 1 minute.
Walk slowly 1 minute.
Repeat 8 times.
Total time: 16 minutes

Week 3
Walk briskly 2 minutes.
Walk slowly 1 minute.
Repeat 5 times, then walk briskly 2 minutes.
Total time: 17 minutes

Week 4
Walk briskly 3 minutes.
Walk slowly 1 minute.
Repeat 4 times.
Total time: 16 minutes

Week 5
Walk briskly 4 minutes.
Walk slowly 1 minute.
Repeat 3 times.
Total time: 15 minutes

Week 6
Walk briskly 5 minutes.
Walk slowly 1 minute.
Repeat 3 times.
Total time: 18 minutes

Week 7
Walk briskly 6 minutes.
Walk slowly 1 minute.
Repeat 2 times, then walk slowly 6 minutes.
Total time: 20 minutes

Week 8
Walk briskly 8 minutes.
Walk slowly 1 minute.
Repeat 2 times.
Total time: 18 minutes

Week 9
Walk briskly 10 minutes.
Walk slowly 1 minute.
Repeat.
Total time: 22 minutes

Week 10
Walk briskly 20 minutes nonstop.
Total time: 20 minutes

*This means walking quickly and moving your arms as you walk.
**This is more of a stroll.

Amazing Walkers

Happy Trails

In 1948, Earl Shaffer was the first person to hike the Appalachian Trail end-to-end. In 1965, he did it again. And, 50 years after his first historic hike, Shaffer completed the 2,150-mile journey once more. This time the 173-day trip traversing 14 states, was completed in $5^{1}/_{2}$ months. At the end of his journey, the 79-year-old walker, toting an Army-issue backpack, was in rare form. Only about 20 percent of the 1,500 people who attempt to hike the Appalachian Trail in its entirety each year actually succeed.

Getting Results

Maybe you're already walking but aren't sure if you're making the most of your routine. All movement is good movement, but to get in shape and see results, you'll need to walk regularly at a brisk pace. Brisk walking is fast and steady, enough to get your pulse up to a fairly high rate. This type of walking is valuable as an aerobic exercise and one in which a gain in strength and power is guaranteed.

How do you know if you're walking fast enough to give your heart a good workout? By determining your *Target Heart Rate,* and then adjusting your walking pace to reach this level. Your Target Heart Rate (THR) is what to aim for while you're exercising. It tells you if you're getting the most out of your physical activity, or if you're working too hard.

"I had a heart attack and bypass surgery in 1995. Since then, I have been a mall walker, and I've walked so many hours that I've won all the incentive prizes the mall offers. It's a great bunch of people. I start talking and just keep walking! It was easy to build up to my current level gradually because there were benches to rest on, water fountains to drink from, and bathrooms everywhere."

EILEEN

Reach Your Target Heart Rate

About halfway through your walk, check your heart rate by taking your pulse. This may require some practice, so first get used to finding your pulse while you're at rest.

You can find your pulse on your wrist and on your neck (on either side of your Adam's apple). Always take your pulse *lightly* with two fingers—not your thumb because your thumb has a pulse, too, and won't give you as accurate a measurement. Count the beats while watching the second hand on your watch, timing yourself for one minute. Tip: When you take your pulse for sixty seconds, your heart rate naturally slows down during this time, so it's not always possible to get the most accurate results. Another way to measure your pulse is to count the number of beats you feel in fifteen seconds, then multiply this number by four. Choose whichever method works best for you.

A resting pulse rate is generally between sixty and eighty beats per minute. Yours may be higher or lower than this. During activity, your pulse rate will vary depending on several factors, including your age, fitness level, intensity of exercise, and certain medications.

Your *maximum heart rate*—the highest rate you can reach safely during your workout—can be determined by subtracting your age from the number 220. Most fitness experts recommend that you aim for 60 to 80 percent of your maximum heart rate while exercising—this is your Target Heart Rate (THR). If you're just starting a walking program, you should stay at the lower end of this range (60 percent).

Follow this simple equation to estimate your Target Heart Rate:

1. Subtract your age from 220 for your maximum heart rate.
2. Multiply your maximum heart rate by 60 percent (0.6) if you're a beginner, or 80 percent (0.8) if you're in better shape. Or try 70 percent (0.7) if you fall somewhere in between.
3. This number is your Target Heart Rate.

Example #1

Age 55

1. 220 - 55 = 165
2. 165 x 0.6 = 99
3. Target Heart Rate is 99

Example #2

Age 35

1. 220 - 35 = 185
2. 185 x 0.8 = 148
3. Target Heart Rate is 148

After about fifteen minutes of brisk walking, take your pulse to find out if you're close to your THR. If your pulse is way above this number, you're walking too fast and you need to slow down. If your pulse is far below it, you can work a little harder by increasing your pace and swinging your arms more. Once you become a regular walker, you should aim to stay at your Target Heart Rate for a minimum of twenty minutes.

"I wear a heart rate monitor to make sure that I'm not walking too fast or too slow—it's as easy as wearing a wristwatch. It shows my heart rate at all times."

DOUG

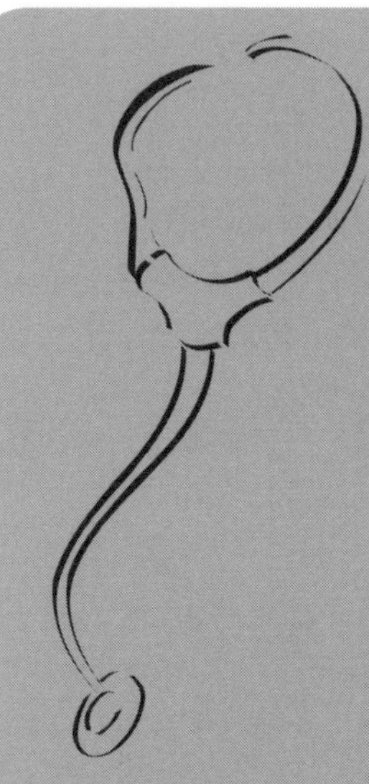

Remember, when it comes to your heart rate, higher isn't necessarily better. Don't think that aiming for your maximum heart rate during your exercise routine will help you reach your fitness goals faster. Moderation is the key. It's best to reach—not exceed—your Target Heart Rate during your walk, and as you become more fit, to increase the length of time you stay at this level.

One last thing: If you're taking medication, talk to your doctor about your THR; some medications slow the resting heart rate, which could affect your calculations. If you have high blood pressure, make sure your doctor knows about your walking program before you start.

Pace Yourself

Once you become a regular walker, gradually increase the frequency, length, and speed of your walks, always maintaining a reasonably comfortable pace. Make it your goal to walk for at least thirty minutes, but preferably forty-five to sixty minutes, at least four days a week. Most of all, enjoy yourself!

Here are a few tips for a successful walk every time:

1. **Stretch before and after you walk.** Stretching loosens your muscles, which allows you to take longer strides and reduces your risk of soreness and injury. See chapter 3, "Flexibility and Stretching: Loosen Up!" for suggested stretches.

2. **Warm up.** Warming up before you walk loosens your joints and muscles, and increases your flexibility. To warm up, march in place, walk at a slow pace, or do some other type of rhythmic movement. Continue for five to ten minutes, giving yourself time to increase your heart rate slowly and safely.

3. **Walk correctly.** Keep an upright posture as you walk. Strike the ground heel-first, roll through to your toes, and allow your toes and the ball of your foot to help push off the next step. Take long, smooth strides—but not so long that you feel uncomfortable. Your knees should be slightly bent.

   Pump your arms to enhance your stride, making sure you're bending your elbows. Your hands should be cupped but relaxed. (This may sound like a lot to remember, but most people walk this way naturally. Just check yourself every so often to be sure you're not letting your arms hang or forgetting to bend your knees.)

4. **Choose a comfortable pace.** Walking shouldn't be painful and exhausting—you should feel energized and in control. Try to reach your THR, adjusting your walking pace as needed to speed up or slow down your heart rate. Experts say the most efficient rate of walking is about 2.4 miles per hour—you can aim for this goal over time.

When you're a regular walker, you'll be able to walk for a longer period at a quicker pace. Remember not to do too much too fast. Listen to your body—it will let you know if you're pushing yourself beyond your limits.

5. Watch your breathing when you exercise. If you're breathing so fast that it's difficult to speak, or if you're short of breath, you're working way too hard. And if you feel pain in your joints, try taking shorter and more frequent walks. Pain and shortness of breath are your body's way of telling you that you're doing too much; stop the exercise and consult your doctor before going any further.

6. Cool down. Don't just go from a brisk walk to a complete standstill. Give your body time to wind down and relax. A cool-down keeps your muscles from tightening up and allows your heart to return to its resting level. To cool down, reduce your speed gradually until you're strolling, then keep going at this rate for at least five minutes. Stretch afterward.

"I walk with different groups of friends different days of the week, depending on how good I feel. Some days are faster than others, and some are slower. Mostly, I just remember to choose a pace that I know I can comfortably walk."

ALICE

Measure Your Progress

According to the American College of Sports Medicine (ACSM), the rate at which your fitness level increases depends on:

- your health
- your age
- your own preferences, needs, and goals

No one can tell you for sure how quickly you'll see the results of your walking program. If you're hoping to lose weight, increase your muscle mass, look younger, and get healthier, keep in mind that these benefits come in time—not right away. The key is sticking with your program long enough to reap these rewards. There is one guarantee, however: Walking regularly will help you *feel* better. After just a couple of weeks, you'll notice that you have more mental and physical energy. Keep it up, and you'll see even bigger results inside and out!

An effective walking program contains three ingredients:

1. **frequency** (how often you walk),
2. **duration** (how long you walk), and
3. **intensity** (how hard you walk).

These three ingredients help create a recipe for success. On the following page, you'll find an explanation of how to put them together.

INGREDIENT #1

The *frequency* of your walks is an important factor in determining your success. Experts say that if you work out three times per week, you can expect noticeable—but not drastic—results in three to six weeks. If you walk less often, your fitness level will improve more slowly (but remember that something is better than nothing!).

Make it your goal to eventually walk four or five times per week, but don't rush it. Some walkers take months, or even years, to reach this level. Tip: Walking more than five times per week may increase your risk of injury. If you walk every day, you can reduce your risk by taking shorter walks or slowing your pace on some days of the week. And don't forget to stretch!

INGREDIENT #2

The *duration* of your walks depends on your fitness level. Continue monitoring your Target Heart Rate to determine whether you're working out at a pace that's right for you. Once you're able to walk briskly for twenty minutes a few times per week, you're ready to increase the duration of your walks—and, as a result, increase your level of aerobic fitness.

Start by extending the duration of one of your walks by fifteen minutes each week, but don't extend the time of your other walks quite yet. When your shorter walks get easier, you can increase the duration of another one of them by fifteen minutes each week. When you're ready, increase the duration of one more shorter walk. Continue this slow and steady increase (there's no need to hurry) until each walk you take is of a longer duration.

INGREDIENT #3

The *intensity* of your walks is up to you. If you're consistently reaching your Target Heart Rate, you're working at the right intensity. You're getting too intense if you can't walk and talk at the same time, or if you're short of breath. You should be perspiring at the end of your walk—not about to collapse.

If you want to increase the intensity of your walks, do so gradually. You can swing your arms harder, walk faster, or even use hand-held weights as you walk. Just be sure you don't exceed your maximum heart rate or exhaust yourself. You don't want to push yourself so hard that you no longer enjoy your walks.

Before you pick up the pace of your exercise routine, take the quiz on the following page. Are you *really* ready to go a little farther or a little faster?

DID YOU KNOW . . .

Walkers are less likely to smoke cigarettes than inactive people.

Walkers are more likely to follow good nutritional habits than inactive people.

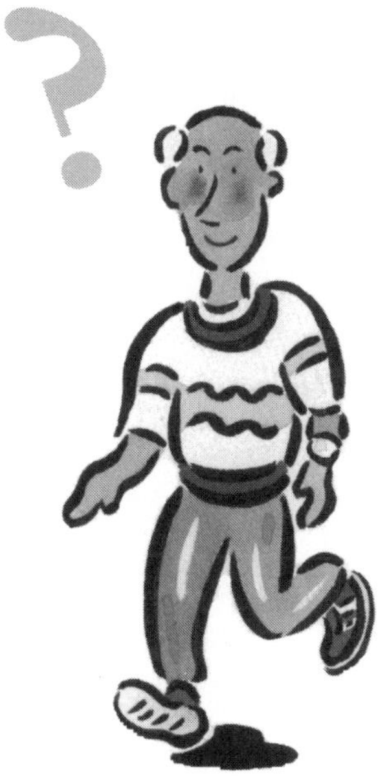

Readiness Quiz

1. Can I walk for twenty to thirty minutes continuously at a constant intensity?

   __ yes __ no

2. Am I healthy and injury free?

   __ yes __ no

3. Do I feel energized by my current walking routine?

   __ yes __ no

4. Am I ready to set new goals and exercise a little longer?

   __ yes __ no

5. Do I recover quickly after an exercise session?

   __ yes __ no

If you answered yes to all of these questions, you're ready to *gradually* increase the frequency, duration, and intensity of your walking routine. To do this safely, focus first on increasing the number of days you walk (frequency). Once you've achieved this goal, you're ready to increase the number of minutes you walk (duration). Finally, you can focus on putting more energy into each walk (intensity). Now you're making progress!

Keep a Journal

Keeping an exercise journal is a great way to track your progress and stay motivated to walk. The following pages contain a sample Exercise Journal that you can photocopy and use each week. There's room to fill out your goals and progress. Keep notes about how long you walked, how you felt, and even what you thought about as you walked, if you'd like. Record any challenges or setbacks you faced. Be sure to list ideas for future fitness goals, too. Store all the filled-out pages in a notebook, so you can review your progress any time.

Your exercise journal is also a good place to collect magazine articles about exercise or athletes you admire, inspirational quotes, nutrition tips, low-fat recipes, and anything else that motivates you. You can even write down positive comments people have made about your commitment to fitness, or compliments you've received about improvements in your appearance.

"My motto is: 'Exercise each day will keep the doctor away.' I started a daily walking program after visiting my doctor for a minor knee problem. He told me to lose weight and strengthen my legs. After a year of walking and losing twenty pounds, I completed my first marathon at age forty-nine by walking 26.2 miles in six hours. It was a wonderful accomplishment!"

ANN

Exercise Journal

For the week of: ________________

My exercise goals:

Sunday:
Monday:
Tuesday:
Wednesday:
Thursday:
Friday:
Saturday:

Exercise log (what I really accomplished):

Sunday:
Monday:
Tuesday:
Wednesday:
Thursday:
Friday:
Saturday:

Did I reach my goals? How did this feel?

Setbacks I faced:

New ideas or goals for next week:

Exercise Journal

For the week of: ________________

My exercise goals:

Sunday:
Monday:
Tuesday:
Wednesday:
Thursday:
Friday:
Saturday:

Exercise log (what I really accomplished):

Sunday:
Monday:
Tuesday:
Wednesday:
Thursday:
Friday:
Saturday:

Did I reach my goals? How did this feel?

Setbacks I faced:

New ideas or goals for next week:

6 *Staying* Cool

"I am a walker. Walking is my hobby, exercise, medicine, and profession. It is my life."

ROBERT SWEETGALL

Your mall walking program is giving you a chance to change your life and improve your health. You're discovering that you can walk away from an inactive lifestyle and become stronger, healthier, and more fit. A key part of this new outlook is knowing this: *Sweat is good for you.* In fact, it's a sign of fitness.

Let Them See You Sweat

You're probably aware that sweating is your body's way of cooling itself in hot weather or during a workout. Sweat is basically water escaping through your sweat glands. When it evaporates from the surface of your skin, you cool down. But you may not know that sweating declines with age. In other words, the older you get the less you sweat.

You can prevent this decline through regular exercise. Studies have shown that older people who exercise a few hours per week improve their ability to sweat and regulate their body temperature. So head to the mall and work up a sweat!

"At one time, I thought sweating wasn't attractive, or something women did. You know that saying about women don't sweat, they glow? That was me. I didn't do much. But now I'm out there sweating with the rest of them. I've lost weight, and I feel great."

MARGE

Cool Down with Water

The American Dietetic Association (ADA) recommends drinking at least eight to twelve glasses of water each day. Does this sound like a lot to you? If so, you may not be drinking enough water. Water is an essential nutrient that keeps your body hydrated and healthy. For optimum health, consider drinking more than the ADA recommendation: Aim for two quarts per day.

Why drink so much? Because water plays a vital role in your body by lubricating your joints and internal organs, carrying nutrients to your cells, regulating your body temperature, and helping eliminate wastes. Water also hydrates your body and skin, helping to keep muscles and skin more supple.

Water has many other virtues such as:

- **Aiding weight loss.** Water doesn't have any calories, and it helps you feel full. It also prevents fluid retention, which causes bloating.
- **Reducing wrinkles.** Well-hydrated skin is smoother and less prone to developing fine wrinkles. In fact, water is probably the best anti-aging "vitamin" for your skin.
- **Flushing your kidneys.** Drinking lots of water flushes your kidneys, which helps your urinary tract better resist bacteria.
- **Helping medications do their work.** If you're on any type of prescription drug, be sure to take it with a full glass of water. Water helps medications dissolve more quickly and be more readily absorbed by your system. In addition, water reduces the stomach irritation caused by some drugs.

"Drinking eight glasses of water per day raises my energy level. I think pop and sugary beverages slow my mind."

BEV

*A*mazing Walkers

Splish, Splash, I Was Takin' a Bath

When Choi Jong Yul jumped into the Red Sea on June 5, 1996, it was a fitting end to a long journey. The 38-year-old South Korean had just become the first person ever to walk across the Sahara Desert. Sweaty and exhausted from the 4,588-mile journey, he jumped fully clothed into the water at the Sudanese port of Suakin. Averaging 40 miles a day, he battled sun, sand, and scorpions to blaze a historic path, west to east, across five countries in seven months. (Thankfully, the Red Sea was no mirage.)

You can drink expensive bottled water or plain tap water—both quench your thirst and hydrate your body. Just don't make the mistake of believing the water in coffee, tea, or juice counts as part of your daily water requirement. These beverages contain caffeine (which acts as a diuretic), sugar, or other chemicals.

A little-known fact of aging is that thirst tends to decline the older you get. When your body doesn't tell you it's thirsty, you may drink less and this can lead to dehydration. Dehydration is dangerous for people of all ages, but especially the elderly, who dehydrate more easily in hot weather or due to illness. Symptoms of dehydration include fatigue, a drop in blood pressure, weakness, and even fainting. (If you experience any of these symptoms, you may need medical attention.)

To avoid these problems, develop healthy "drinking habits." Don't wait until you're thirsty to drink. Instead, get into the habit of always keeping a glass or bottle of water within reach and take sips from it throughout the day. You'll feel hydrated and refreshed.

"I like to drink a glass of water before and after my walk. Sometimes I also have a piece of fruit afterward."

MARTY

Water and Your Workouts

The ADA further recommends drinking one to three cups of water per hour during exercise. And the more you sweat, the more water you'll need.

What happens when you *don't* drink water during a workout? Your muscles aren't properly hydrated, which can make you feel tired, weak, and uncoordinated. Your best bet is to drink some water before, during, and after exercising. Carry along a water bottle when you walk, or memorize where in the mall the water fountains are located. Staying hydrated will allow you to put more energy into each step.

DID YOU KNOW . . .

To survive, all living things need the same concentration of water in their body. A healthy adult is 60 to 65 percent water by weight—as is the largest elephant and the tiniest mouse!

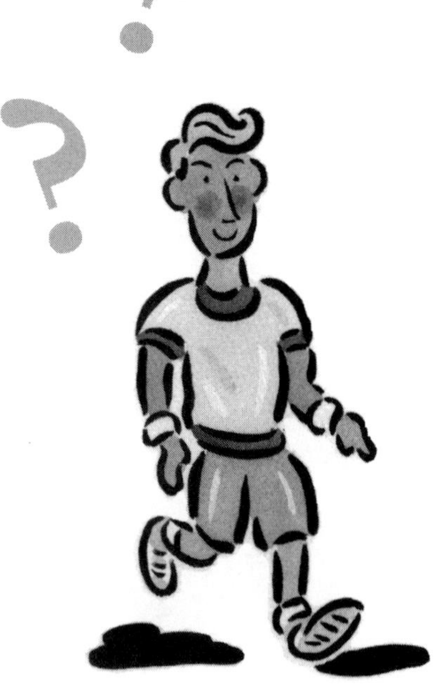

*A*mazing WALKERS

One Step at a Time

When James J. Johnson proclaimed golf was good exercise, he wasn't kidding. In October of 1959, Johnson became the first golfer to walk continuously for 24 hours on the 6,101-yard Abilene Country Club golf course in Fort Worth, Texas. Johnson played 363 holes over a two-day period. Historians may never remember his golf score, but his walking feat is one for the history books.

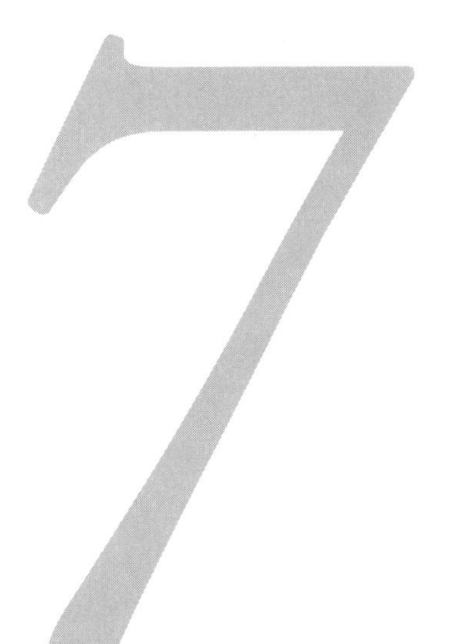

7 *Eat Right for* Life

"Your body is the baggage you must carry through life. The more excess baggage, the shorter the trip."
ARNOLD H. GLASOW

Your body is your own personal vehicle that takes you from place to place. And to keep it running smoothly and efficiently, you need to give it the proper fuel: healthy food. This probably isn't the first time you've read something about the importance of good nutrition. But did you know that eating right—starting now—decreases your risk of certain health problems (like heart disease, osteoporosis, some forms of cancer, stroke, and diabetes)? And makes you leaner? And gives you the energy to stick with your walking program?

There are so many good reasons to pay attention to what you eat. Eating a balanced diet improves your health by providing the vitamins and nutrients you need, helping you control your weight, keeping your heart in better shape, and reducing your risk of chronic disease. When you eat right, you feel better and you have a more positive outlook on life.

The U.S. Department of Agriculture (USDA) and the U.S. Department of Health and Human Services (USDHHS) have created the *Dietary Guidelines for Americans* and the Food Guide Pyramid to encourage people of all ages to eat right and understand the benefits of nutrition. Together, the guidelines and pyramid offer an easy, practical way to improve your diet. Even if your schedule is hectic, you can use these tools to put healthy eating into practice.

Attention SHOPPERS!

The first climate-controlled suburban shopping mall was Southdale, located in Edina, a suburb of Minneapolis, Minnesota. Designed by Victor Gruen in 1956, this mall boasted two shopping levels and a garden court. This innovation is now a familiar sight in suburban malls nationwide.

Dietary Guidelines for Americans

How would you rate your own eating habits? Healthy? Not-so-healthy? Unhealthy? If you're on the lower end of this rating scale (you eat a poor diet), it's time to make some changes. You have the power to be more productive at home and at work, and to feel your best, by changing your diet. And this doesn't mean *going on a diet.* Even if your goal is to lose weight, depriving yourself of food isn't the answer. Instead, you can focus on choosing foods that are nutrient-dense and low in fat. This way, you're eating more of the foods that promote health and prevent disease.

According to the *Dietary Guidelines for Americans,* here are seven simple steps you can take to improve your eating habits:

1. Eat a variety of foods. Many of us fall into a food rut. We eat the same old breakfast every morning, buy the same sandwich for lunch, and have a standard set of menus we prepare for our family dinners. Because our bodies need many different nutrients for good health, it's important to consume different foods during every meal, every day. Choose a variety of fruits, vegetables, grains, dairy products, meats, fish, dry beans and other legumes, eggs, nuts, rice, and pasta.

2. Balance the food you eat with physical activity—maintain or improve your weight. An active lifestyle keeps you strong and fit. You burn more calories, build more muscle, and lose fat. The more active you are, the more efficient your body becomes at burning calories—even when you're resting! It's a win-win proposition.

"My friend and I used to walk around the lake once and then go for coffee. Now our endurance is better, so we walk the lake twice. We catch up on our chatting even more, and we do not miss the donuts."

ROSE

3. Choose a diet with plenty of whole grain products, vegetables, and fruits. These foods are rich in vitamins, minerals, complex carbohydrates, and fiber—all of which your body needs for optimum health. Fruits, in particular, are loaded with vitamin C, and vegetables provide a variety of vitamins (especially A and C). These foods also give you energy and are naturally low in fat. Make it your goal to eat more fresh and dried fruits each day, and avoid fruit processed with heavy syrups and sugar-sweetened juices. For maximum nutrients, choose orange or yellow vegetables; dark, leafy greens; and starchy vegetables like potatoes.

4. Choose a diet low in fat, saturated fat, and cholesterol. A diet high in fat increases your risk of obesity, heart disease, and some forms of cancer, so it's best to watch your fat intake. The same goes for a diet high in cholesterol. In addition, foods high in fat, saturated fat, and cholesterol usually aren't nutritious—they provide few vitamins and minerals, and they aren't a good source of fiber. You can cut your fat and cholesterol intake by reducing the amount of potato chips, dips, sweets, red meat, creamy sauces, butter, mayonnaise, and high-fat cheeses you consume on a daily basis.

5. Choose a diet moderate in sugars. Most of us aren't even aware that we consume too much sugar. This is because sugar is hidden in many of the packaged foods we eat every day: salad dressing, yogurt, lunch meats, canned sauces, frozen dinners, and peanut butter. Other foods are a more obvious source of sugar: muffins, cookies, brownies, ice cream, sodas, and sweet rolls. All of this sugar adds up to extra calories. And when you fill up on soft drinks and sugary treats, you may end up eating less of the healthy foods your body needs. To cut down on sugar, buy fewer sweets when you're at the grocery store, switch to sugar-free sodas and gum, and consume less packaged foods.

6. Choose a diet moderate in salt and sodium. Your doctor might have told you that too much salt and sodium in your diet increases your risk of high blood pressure, stroke, or heart disease. But you may not realize how much you're actually consuming each day. Like sugar, sodium is added to many packaged foods like margarine, soups, pasta sauces, and frozen meals (this helps preserve the foods and make them taste better). People who consume a lot of sodium learn to crave it in the foods they eat. If you crave salt and sodium, reduce your intake gradually. Eat fewer packaged/processed foods, eliminate fast foods from your diet, and put "light" salt in the salt shaker.

7. If you drink alcoholic beverages, do so in moderation. Consumption of alcohol has been linked to high blood pressure, stroke, some forms of cancer, and liver and kidney problems. The guidelines recommend that women drink no more than one alcoholic beverage per day, and men no more than two.

When you're walking at the mall and feel like going out for a snack afterward, remind yourself of the seven dietary guidelines. It's always tempting to reach for sweets or "reward" yourself with your favorite fast-food treat, but keep in mind all the good things you're doing for your body when you walk. Instead of buying food that's high in fat, sugar, or sodium, go for a snack that's healthy and tasty. With a wide array of restaurants and food stands at the mall, it shouldn't be hard to find salads, low-fat frozen yogurt, fruit smoothies, or other healthy snacks that taste good, fill you up, and make you feel like you're treating your body well.

The Food Guide Pyramid

You don't have to hire a dietitian or become a nutrition expert yourself to figure out if you're eating right. You can use the Food Guide Pyramid, a tool developed by food and health experts who spent years doing all the research for you. The pyramid—which is recommended by every major health and scientific organization in the U.S. as an excellent way to develop a healthy diet—offers you an easy way to eat right for life.

Each day, try to improve your eating habits using the pyramid as a guide. Here's an explanation of how it works:

LEVEL 1: This level is made up of the Bread, Cereal, Rice, and Pasta Group. You should eat 6–11 servings from this group each day. (Servings = 1 slice of bread, 1/2 cup cooked rice, 1 oz. breakfast cereal, 1/2 cup cooked pasta, or 1/2 bagel.)

LEVEL 2: This level includes both the Fruit Group and the Vegetable Group. The USDA recommends that you eat at least 3–5 servings of vegetables and 2–4 servings of fruit each day. (Servings = 1 medium piece of fresh fruit, 1 cup canned fruit, or 6 oz. fruit juice; 1 cup raw, leafy greens, 1/2 cup chopped or cooked vegetables, or 3/4 cup vegetable juice.)

LEVEL 3: This level consists of the Milk, Yogurt, and Cheese Group and the Meat, Fish, Poultry, Dry Beans, Eggs, and Nuts Group. The daily goal is to eat 2–3 servings from the first group and 2–3 servings from the second. (Servings = 1 cup milk or yogurt, 2 cups cottage cheese, 1 oz. cheese; 3 eggs, 1 cup cooked beans, 3 oz. cooked meat/poultry/fish, or 1 cup nuts.)

LEVEL 4: This level features Fats, Oils, and Sweets—foods to cut down on. Consume them sparingly.

The Food Guide Pyramid

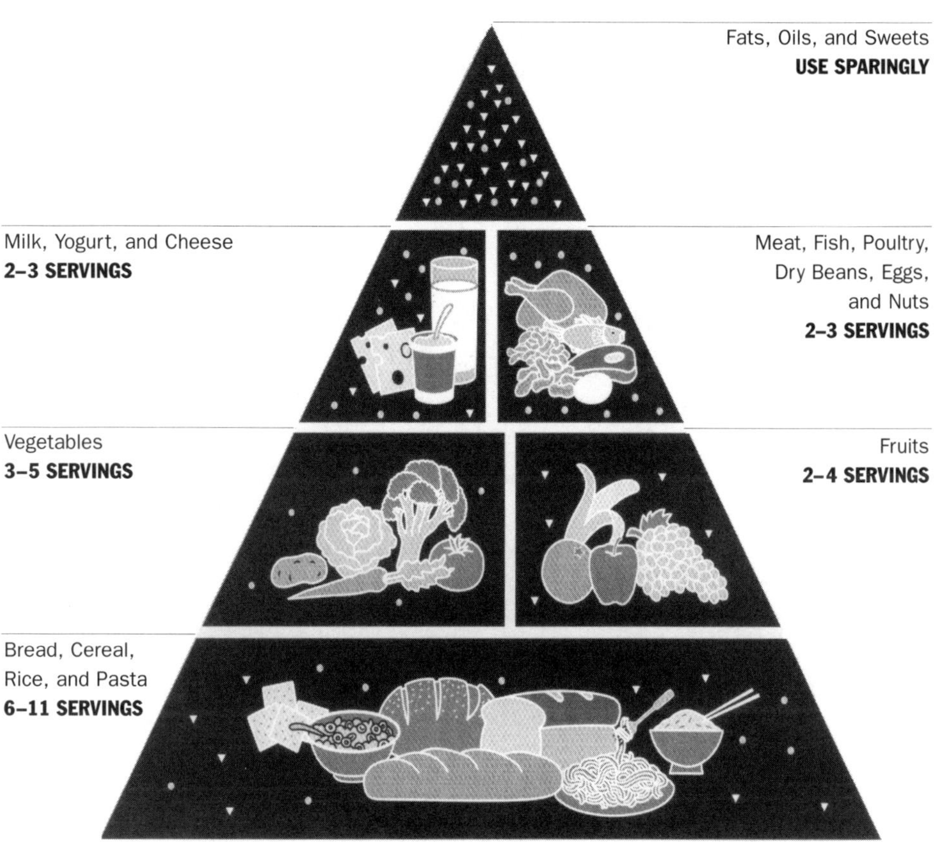

U.S. Department of Agriculture/U.S. Department of Health and Human Services

■ Fat (naturally occurring and added)

▼ Sugars (added)

These symbols show that fat and added sugars come mostly from fats, oils, and sweets, but can be part of or added to foods from the other food groups as well.

If You're over Age Seventy

Recently, experts at the Human Nutrition Research Center on Aging at Tufts University in Boston studied the effects of diet on older Americans, whose nutritional needs change as they age. As a result of these studies, a new pyramid was developed which specifically addresses the dietary needs of people ages seventy and older. (The pyramid appears on page 114.) It's similar to the standard Food Guide Pyramid but includes five levels, with a special emphasis on the need for water and vitamin supplements.

Here's an explanation of how the five-level pyramid works:

LEVEL 1: The base of the pyramid includes a recommendation to drink water, specifically 8 servings a day or more. For more information about the importance of water, see chapter 6, "Staying Cool."

"I carry a water bottle with me wherever I go—not just when I'm doing my exercise."

SALLY

LEVEL 2: This level features the Bread, Fortified Cereal, Rice, and Pasta Group. Eat 6 or more servings from this group each day, making sure you choose fiber-rich and vitamin-fortified options like whole-grain breads and cereals. (Servings = 1 slice of wheat bread, 1/2 cup cooked rice, 1 oz. fortified breakfast cereal, 1/2 cup cooked pasta, or 1/2 wheat bagel.)

LEVEL 3: This level includes both the Fruit Group and the Vegetable Group. Consume 2 or more servings of actual fruit (not juices) and 3 or more servings of richly colored vegetables each day. (Servings = 1 medium piece of fresh fruit or 1 cup canned fruit without heavy syrup; 1 cup raw, leafy greens or 1/2 cup chopped or cooked vegetables.)

LEVEL 4: This level consists of the Milk, Yogurt, and Cheese Group and the Meat, Poultry, Fish, Dry Beans, Eggs, and Nut Group. The daily goal is to eat 3 or more low-fat servings from the first group and 2 or more servings from the second, with an emphasis on consuming fish, dried beans with lots of fiber, and lean cuts of meat. (Servings = 1 cup low-fat milk or yogurt, 2 cups low-fat cottage cheese, 1 oz. low-fat cheese; 3 eggs, 1 cup cooked beans, 3 oz. cooked meat/poultry/fish, or 1 cup nuts.)

LEVEL 5: This level features Fats, Oils, and Sweets—foods to cut down on.

An added feature is the "flag" at the top of the pyramid, which alerts people over seventy to the need for calcium, vitamin D, and vitamin B-12 supplements. Talk to your doctor about the amount of vitamins you should be taking each day.

Modified Food Pyramid for 70+ Adults

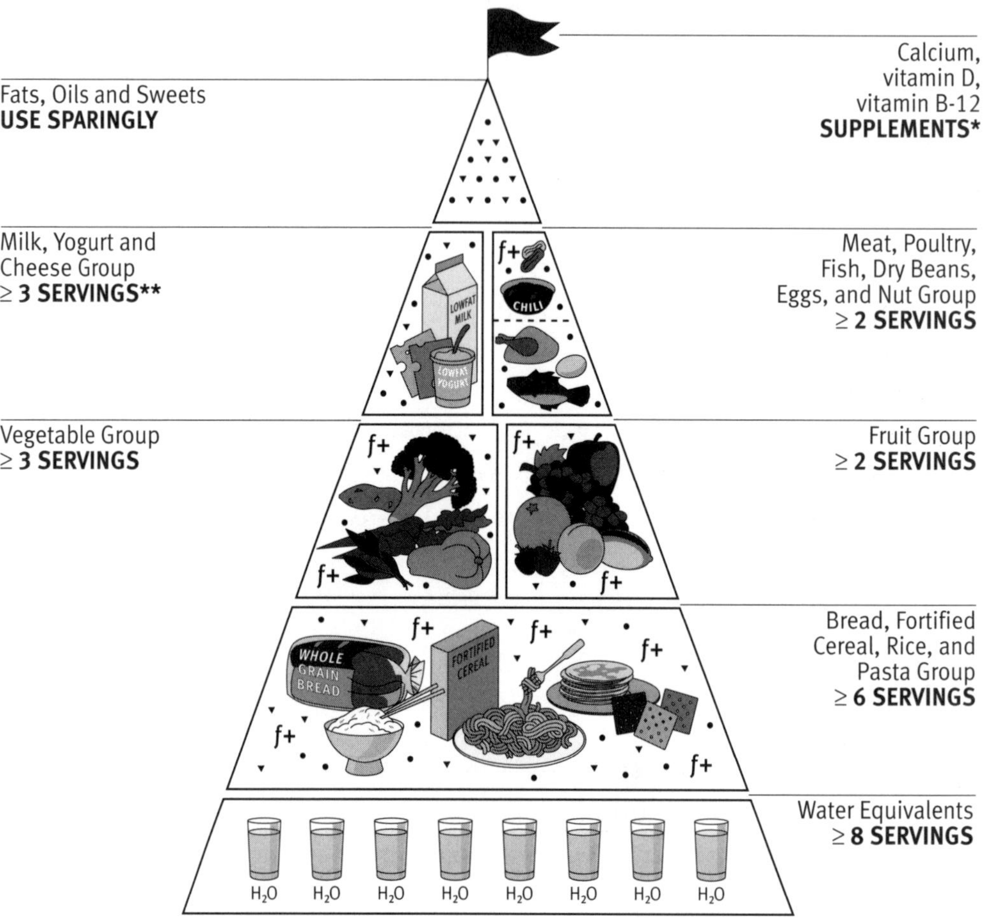

● **Fat** (naturally occuring and added)

▼ **Sugars** (added)

f+ **Fiber** (should be present)

These symbols show fat, added sugars, and fiber in foods

*Not all individuals need supplements, consult your healthcare provider

** ≥ Greater than or equal to

Get accustomed to using the pyramid (whichever one is appropriate for your age) by keeping a log of the foods you eat for a week or two. Write down what you ate, how much, and when you ate it, and be sure to note the portion size. Then compare your log to the pyramid's recommended number of daily servings. Are you eating a balanced diet and choosing a variety of foods from all but the "fats" level? Are you skipping meals? Snacking a lot? Eating too much from the tip of the pyramid?

As an alternative, keep your food log but also draw a picture of the pyramid (it doesn't have to be detailed), dividing up the levels and noting the name of each group. At the end of the day, tally up the foods you've consumed, putting check marks (representing servings you've eaten) in each corresponding level/group of the pyramid. Do you have 3–5 check marks in the Vegetable Group? Do you have 2–3 check marks in the Milk, Yogurt, and Cheese Group? Do you have too many check marks under Fats, Oils, and Sweets? Too few in the Bread, Cereal, Rice, and Pasta Group?

Decide where you need to make changes, then get started. If you have specific questions about your diet, talk to your doctor or consult a registered dietitian in your area by contacting the American Dietetic Association's Nationwide Nutrition Network (1-800-366-1655, Monday–Friday, 10 A.M.–5 P.M. EST; *http://www.eatright.org/finddiet.html*).

You may want to ask your spouse or other family members to join you in your commitment to eating right. It's easier to stay focused and motivated when you have your family's support.

8 *Tips for* Mall Walkers

"Mall walking is one of the best things you can do. I walk three to four times a week and have a card that keeps track of the number of hours I've walked. It's amazing how many of my neighbors I see here. People come here for the social benefits."

DUANE

Most mall walkers choose a mall and walk at that one on a regular basis. Other mall walkers like to vary their routine by exercising at different local malls. You can do whatever works for you, depending on what's available in your community.

Some of the larger malls nationwide have mall-walking programs that draw large numbers of walkers. Highlights of these programs may include:

- early-morning hours for mall walkers
- informational seminars on heart health, exercise, safety, nutrition, and other topics
- monthly activities sponsored by a local hospital or other healthcare organization
- free blood pressure checks, cholesterol tests, body-fat measuring, and other diagnostic screenings
- educational speakers and presenters
- demonstrations of proper walking techniques
- membership cards
- special incentives for mall walkers (prizes, coupons, store discounts, and so forth)
- computerized cards that record the miles or hours you've walked, or even the approximate number of calories you've burned
- maps that indicate the distance around the mall at each level, so you can track your progress

"People come to walk at the mall for the social aspect. There is also free coffee for senior citizens."

GARY

If your local mall has perks like this, take advantage of them! This is a great way to make the most of your mall-walking experience. Plus, you can get to know other mall walkers and even make new friends.

Be sure to show your support for the program and let the sponsors know what's working. Give them feedback about the speakers, special events, incentives, and so on. Offer comments about the program newsletter, if there is one, and ideas for new articles. If your mall-walking program features a suggestion box, make use of it. If there's no suggestion box, suggest one!

Attention SHOPPERS!

The first pedestrian shopping mall was created in 1959 along a section of Burdick Street in downtown Kalamazoo, Michigan. The shopping concept, aimed at preserving the downtown shopping area, earned Kalamazoo the royal title of "Mall City, USA." Unfortunately, shoppers still flocked to the princely new suburban malls, turning downtown retailing into a pauper's paradise.

Promoting a Walking Program at Your Local Mall

If your mall doesn't have a walking program, consider talking to the mall's management staff to find out why. Some malls don't want to be responsible for possible injuries, and if this is the case, suggest that the staff develop a consent form mall walkers must sign before joining the program. Perhaps the mall staff isn't aware of how much public support there might be for a mall-walking program. If you have friends, neighbors, and coworkers who want to mall walk, ask them to call the promotions department of the mall to express their interest.

You may even want to volunteer your time to get the program underway. You could help the mall create a mission statement for the program and come up with goals and objectives to meet this mission. Or you could help spread the word about the program. Place ads in local newspapers, in community newsletters, or on the radio. Hang colorful posters in churches, health clubs, grocery stores, senior citizen centers, community centers, banks, and hospitals. Come up with a special program name and logo that communicates the physical and social benefits of mall walking.

"I started walking the day the mall opened and come daily in the winter. I am known as 'the mayor' of the mall, and I've won the Mall Walker of the Year award."

LES

Once the program is in place, stay involved—not just by walking but by suggesting new ideas for keeping the program fresh and fun. Ask merchants in the mall to donate items as prizes to mall walkers who complete a designated distance. Popular prizes include:

- water bottles
- books
- mugs
- fanny packs
- gift certificates
- pens and pencils
- T-shirts with the program's logo
- store discounts

"There are so many perks when you're a member, and it's fun to see how many prizes you can get. I've won a fanny pack, a pin, store discounts, a T-shirt, and even tickets to a show in town."

MARTHA

In addition, you may be able to find restaurants that will provide free coffee or juice to mall walkers, or coupons for food items. Another fun incentive is to recognize the individual achievements of walkers involved in the program: Ask the mall to post or announce names of people who have walked a certain number of miles.

Having Fun While You Walk

One of the most important things to remember about mall walking is this: Have fun! You're more likely to keep walking if you look forward to it, enjoy it, and can find creative ways to stay entertained.

Here are some tips for making your mall-walking routine more enjoyable:

1. **Walk with a buddy.** Bring along a friend or meet up with one at the mall. Just make sure you're both at a similar fitness level and can walk at the same pace for the same amount of time. (Family members make good walking buddies, too.)

"The incentive prizes are nice, but I walk to see my friends and stay active with others."

DON

2. **Window shop.** Mall walking is a great way to keep an eye out for bargains—especially if you're at the mall several times a week. Walk by your favorite stores regularly to see what's on sale.

3. **Listen to "walking songs."** Make a cassette tape of tunes that have "walking" or "walk" in the title or chorus—it's a great motivator. Or just listen to music that moves you. (Many malls play music during mall-walking hours, which is enjoyable *if* you like what they play.)

4. **Make plans for after your walk.** You'll be even more motivated if you have something special to look forward to such as coffee with friends, a breakfast or lunch date, or shopping at all the stores you've passed while walking.

5. **Aim for the prizes.** If your mall-walking program includes incentives for miles and/or hours walked, make it your goal to win a prize—then another, and another.

6. Play games. Remember the Alphabet Game during long family car trips? You can play it while mall walking. Look at signs throughout the mall, watching for words that begin with each letter of the alphabet. Once you've found one letter, move on to the next, and the next. You can also create your own mall-walking version of I Spy, or invent other "mind games."

7. Set personal goals. Decide when and how to increase the frequency, duration, or intensity of your walks, then go for it! It may help to keep a journal of your successes, so you can see how much you've accomplished. Get creative with goal-setting. For example, you could figure out the distance to a travel destination (a weekend getaway, a bed-and-breakfast), then reward yourself with a trip to that place once you've walked the number of miles it would take to get there.

8. Enjoy the scenery. Many malls have attractive decorations and store displays, especially during the holiday season. Malls are also a fun place to "people watch." You'll probably see lots of familiar faces if you're a regular mall walker. Wave, say hi, or catch up with someone you know.

9. Think, dream, and plan. Use this time to clear your head. Don't fall into the trap of thinking about all the things you have to do at work or everything you need to catch up on at home. This is your time—dream about your summer garden, imagine a trip you'd like to take, plan a great meal for you and someone special, or just think about wonderful things you'd like to accomplish in the future.

10. Reward yourself. Give yourself a reward for walking—you've earned it. Stop for a fruit smoothie or low-fat yogurt, buy a new sweatshirt, get a massage, or take a hot bath when you get home. These small indulgences not only will remind you that you're doing something positive for yourself but also will help motivate you to stick with your program.

9 Safe Steps

"Your mobility is the next most important asset after your wits, so be aggressive in guarding it, promoting it, protecting it, and extending it."

ALEX COMFORT

*W*alking is easier on your body than many other forms of exercise, so you should be able to walk without worrying too much about hurting yourself. And mall walking is generally safe because the walking surface is smooth, even, and stable. Even so, injuries do sometimes occur. Always take precautions when you walk.

Here are a few reminders for taking safe steps:

- Follow a regular exercise plan to increase your fitness level.
- Do a variety of activities that work different muscles on different days—this will give your body an "active" rest.
- Stretch before and after your walk.
- Include a warm-up and cool-down as part of your walking routine.
- Wear appropriate walking shoes.
- Progress slowly when beginning a walking program or when increasing the intensity of your routine.
- Drink lots of water before, during, and after your walk.
- Remember to keep breathing throughout your walk—don't hold your breath.
- Walk correctly—don't take giant steps or forget to bend your knees.
- Set a pace you can handle.
- Don't push yourself too hard.
- Take good care of yourself by eating right and exercising regularly.
- Keep a journal about how you feel during and after each walk.

Commonsense cautions:

- Don't walk if you feel ill.
- Don't walk if you have a pulled muscle, sprain, strain, or other injury.
- Don't walk after a full meal or with a totally empty stomach.
- Don't compare yourself to others or attempt to match a pace that's too fast. Exercise at a level that feels good to you.

DID YOU KNOW . . .

Ever hear of a walking "leaf?" The East Indian walking leaf is a bright green, three-inch-long insect that looks just like a leaf—that is, until it walks away from you!

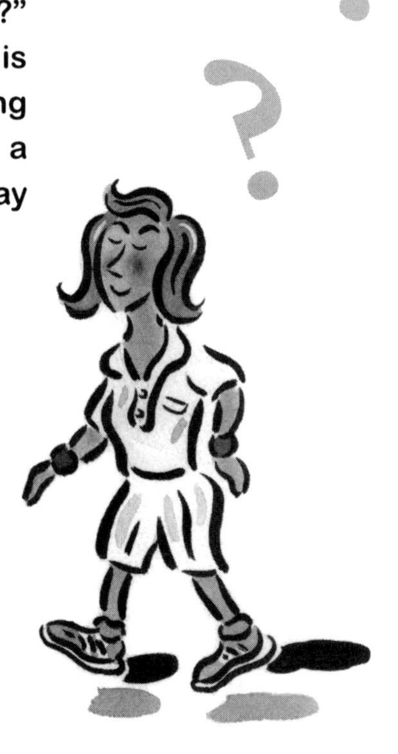

Attention SHOPPERS!

The 4.2 million-square-foot Mall of America, located in Bloomington, Minnesota, opened its doors in 1992 to 35 million visitors in its first year of operation. Shoppers averaged three hours per visit that first year, generating more than $600 million in sales, much of it from tourists.

The Mall of America isn't as big as the 5.2 million-square-foot West Edmonton Mall in Canada, but it's big all right. The Mall of America is 77 football fields of enclosed space with 44 escalators, nearly 13,000 parking spaces, 2.9 miles of hallway, and more than 100 surveillance cameras. One hundred thousand visitors walk the halls daily, seeking exercise, entertainment, food, and a mind-boggling variety of goods.

The 78-acre Mall of America employs around 10,000 people in 400 stores and numerous restaurants and entertainment venues. The parking ramps are the largest in the world, prompting Mall officials to claim that they could accommodate 20 St. Peter's Basilicas. Some say just walking from your car to the mall is a good workout.

Warning Signs

Listen to your body when you walk. Do you feel good, energized, and refreshed? Or tired, run-down, and stressed? Do you have aches and pains? Sore feet? Any other problems? If you do, try to pinpoint where and why you hurt.

Sore feet may be a sign of poor or worn-out walking shoes—something that can easily be fixed. But aches and pains could indicate something more serious. Stop walking for a day or two and see if the pain persists. It helps to keep a journal of how you feel when you walk and at other times, so you have a written record of any problems you're experiencing.

Although some muscle soreness is normal when you first start an exercise program, the pain should only last a couple of days. Similarly, when you increase the duration or intensity of your walks, you might have some minor muscle aches—these, too, should only last a couple of days. If you experience severe pain in your bones, joints, or muscles while walking, this could be a sign of an injury or other health problem. Talk to your doctor—the sooner you get help, the better.

Consult your doctor if you experience any of the following symptoms:

- tenderness in your joints
- swelling or discoloration of your joints
- muscle weakness, stiffness, or tenderness
- persistent muscle soreness
- pain in your knees, tightness of the muscles in your lower legs, or tenderness around your knees
- chest pain
- an aching back
- decline in performance or in daily activities
- chronic fatigue
- dizziness
- nausea
- excessive thirst
- severe weight loss
- loss of appetite
- decreased immunity (more colds or infections than usual)

These symptoms could indicate you're exercising too hard, or they may be a sign of an illness.

Remember, pain shouldn't be a part of your exercise routine. Major aches, soreness, exhaustion, and other physical woes are signals from your body—signals that can't be ignored. Pay attention to what your body is telling you, and walking can continue to be a safe, fun, and rewarding exercise for you.

Amazing Walkers

A Walk That Made History

Thirty-two-year-old historian Anthony Cohen researched and wrote about the Underground Railroad, the life-threatening journey that runaway slaves took to make their escape to Canada. Here they claimed their freedom from the slavery-oppressed United States of the 1800s. Wanting to follow in the footsteps of his ancestors, Cohen planned a walk of 1,000 miles. In 1996, he left Sandy Spring, Maryland, on his solitary trek, with a day's supply of food, a change of clothing, a medicine kit, maps, and an ancient Ethiopian walking stick. Like his forefathers, he found lodging along the way, boarding with sympathetic homeowners and newfound friends eager to help the twentieth-century "fugitive." At the end of his two-month journey, Cohen arrived in Ambertsburg, Ontario, where he was met by the town crier proclaiming, "The town of Ambertsburg welcomes Anthony Cohen—a free man."

10 *Setting Realistic Goals &* Reaching Them

"The sum of the whole is this: walk and be happy; walk and be healthy. The best way to lengthen our days is to walk steadily and with a purpose."
CHARLES DICKENS

*Y*ou've probably set goals for yourself all your life. As a child, you may have saved your allowance for a special toy. In school, you may have tried to achieve a certain grade or challenged yourself to excel in a sport. As a parent, you may have vowed to spend more time with your children. And, like most people, you probably don't let a New Year's Eve go by without setting new goals—resolving to lose weight, exercise regularly, take a fun vacation, get better organized, or spend more time with friends.

Making a pledge is the easy part. Keeping a pledge is a lot tougher. As a mall walker, you've already made a commitment to walk on a regular basis. But how do you keep your resolve? The answer: good goal setting.

DID YOU KNOW . . .

Believe it or not, there is such thing as a walking fish. Florida's walking catfish is capable of moving over land from one body of water to another. They manage this strange walking feat by pushing along the ground with their tail and using their muscular pectoral fins to lift the front of their body. Introduced into Florida from tropical Asian waters in the 1960s, the walking catfish population has flourished.

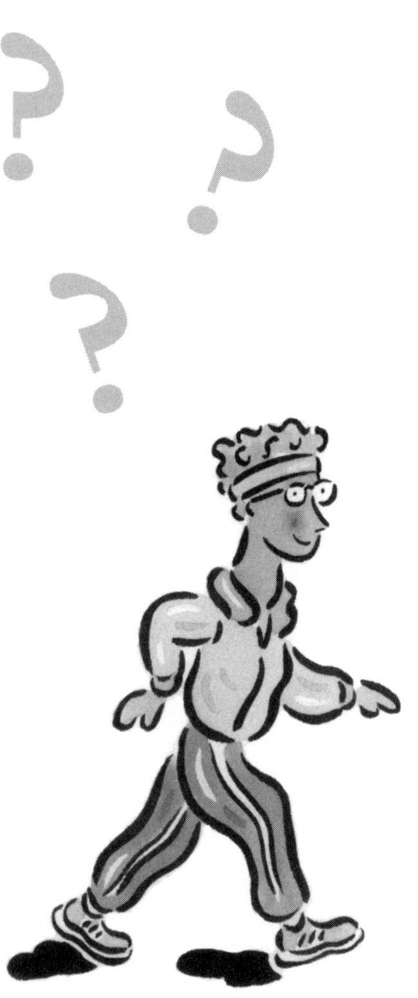

Why Set Goals?

Goals help set direction for your activity. They help you describe what you hope to accomplish by walking. They provide a sense of purpose. And they help you chart your progress.

Would you get on a bus if you had no idea where it was going? Probably not. Then why would you start a mall-walking program without establishing your goals? (If you're already *on* the bus, or in the mall-walking program, you'll still need some direction: Goals provide this direction and help you stay on track.) Think of your goals as stepping stones in your path to success.

Walking just for the sake of walking isn't a goal. An effective goal describes an accomplishment you want to achieve, such as improving your health or losing weight. Your goal should:

- **Be measurable and have an action verb.** ("I want to lose 25 pounds.")
- **Have a time frame.** ("I want to lose 25 pounds in a year.")
- **Include a specific plan of action.** ("I want to lose 25 pounds in one year by walking for 30 minutes at a brisk pace five days a week.")
- **Fit your budget.** (Identify relevant costs like walking shoes, appropriate clothing, and so on.)

Once you've identified these elements, your goal will be more specific and meaningful. You'll know what you want to do and why you want to do it. Now you've taken the first step in goal setting.

Seven Tips to Help You Succeed

Following are seven ways to make your goal an important part of your daily life.

1. Put it in writing. Put your goal on paper and post it where you'll see it each day—your bathroom mirror, the closet door, or the refrigerator.

2. Give it the "sniff test." Once you've written down your goal, take a good, hard look at it. Some goals are real stinkers—they couldn't pass the sniff test. To see if your goal is a good one, ask yourself the following questions: Is it realistic? Does it really fit my schedule? What barriers stand in my way? How can I get past them? Am I being overly ambitious? Is my goal challenging enough? Will it improve my life? If your goal is starting to smell, rewrite it.

3. Chart your course. Keep a monthly calendar near your written goal and mark each day that you make progress. Did you walk today? Give yourself a gold star or bright red check mark. Use your calendar as a visual reminder of the number of days you walk each week.

4. Celebrate your success. Did you walk several days a week during the first month of your walking program? Don't let your progress go unnoticed. Brag to your spouse. Call up a good friend and share your success. Treat yourself to something special.

"When my friend and I walked a total of 300 miles, we treated ourselves to a trip to Las Vegas. We had a blast and walked even more miles on our trip."

VI

5. Value it. Make sure your goal is something you truly value. If the goal is something someone else (your doctor, your spouse) says you should do, it will be harder for you to maintain your resolve. *You* have to want it, too. If you don't value the goal, ask yourself why. Identifying an obstacle is the first step toward overcoming it.

6. Ask for help. Any pledge is easier when you have help. Ask someone to walk with you or join a walking club. Seek encouragement from people you respect—your family members, doctor, spiritual advisor, or a close friend.

7. Envision it. Any goal is more exciting if you can actually imagine it. Try to engage all your senses as you envision your goal. Close your eyes and conjure up a vivid picture of yourself once you've achieved your goal. For example, imagine how you'll look after you've lost 25 pounds. Feel how your clothes will fit you. Experience the renewed energy you'll have. Imagine how easy and brisk your walking pace will be. Hear the compliment from the friend who hasn't seen you for a while. Keep these images in mind as you work toward your goal.

"My doctor recommended exercise, and I agreed it would help me feel better. My health has improved from mall walking three to four times a week. I've belonged to the mall's walking program for six years. I regularly attend monthly meetings to keep motivated."

ED

Getting Back on Track

No matter how much you want to achieve your goals, you may lose your conviction at some point. It can happen to anyone. It's easy to get distracted by responsibilities at work or at home. Or to get discouraged by a lack of progress. Or simply to lose focus.

If this happens to you, don't waste time blaming or criticizing yourself. And don't assume you're a failure and abandon your program altogether. (You've come too far to stop now!) Instead, reassess your situation and find positive ways to recommit to your goal. Here are some tips for getting back on track:

- **Re-evaluate your goal.** Was it too difficult? Not specific enough? Does it need to be revised? What do you need to make it happen?
- **Gain insight from your chart.** Look at your chart or calendar and assess where you've gone astray. Are there certain days of the week when you never walk? If so, what are the reasons and what can you do about them? When did you start to walk less? What happened, and is it something you can change or fix?
- **Think positive.** Spend time recreating the image of yourself reaching your goal. Can you rejuvenate yourself? Don't use setbacks as an excuse to quit.
- **Develop a new plan of action.** Be honest with yourself about why you've slowed down. To help create an action plan, take a piece of paper and make two columns. In the left-hand column, write a list of everything that threw you off course. In the right-hand column, identify one positive step you can take to combat each problem. Take the first step!

Amazing Walkers

No Ordinary Walker

Senior citizen Matt Mattingly decided to take a walk. In 1990, he walked from New York City to San Francisco, a distance of 3,507 miles, in just four months. It was, as he later described it, "a long hot summer and a long walk home."

Six years later, after celebrating his 66th birthday, Mattingly ventured on another walk: This time he walked 2,300 miles from the southern tip of Alaska to his home in Sonora, California, a journey that took him through British Columbia, Washington, Oregon, and California. Of his journey, Mattingly said: "I was a lousy engineer, a terrible manager, a ghastly teacher, an acceptable real estate person, and a reasonable entrepreneur, but I'm a great walker. Most people in life never find something they are good at and something they really enjoy. I have. I am able to walk and I enjoy walking. I consider that I am a success in life."

Amazing Walkers

A Wrong Righted

Everyone thought Ffyona Campbell was the first woman to walk around the world. She began her 11-year journey in Scotland at the age of 16 and reached her goal 19,586 miles later. But, truth be told, the 25-mile-a-day goal she set for herself proved too difficult and she hopped on a van and skipped a few miles during her travels across the United States. The fib festered, and Campbell survived a suicide attempt and drug addiction before confessing that she had cheated along the way. One year after completing her global expedition, Campbell returned to the U.S. to retrace her steps and completed the 1,000 miles she had missed.

On the following page is a form that you can copy and fill out. It's designed to help you pinpoint your goal and find ways to reach it. Every time you reach a goal, set a new one. (You can reuse the form any time you're ready to take on another challenge.)

Henry Ford once said, "Whether you think you can or you think you can't, you're right." Positive thinking plus clear, measurable goals is a powerful combination that can lead you down the path to a rewarding mall-walking program and to better health.

Attention SHOPPERS!

West Edmonton Mall in Alberta, Canada, is often called the "Eighth Wonder of the World." Covering 48 city blocks or the equivalent of 115 football fields, it is the world's largest mall. This amazing structure contains 26 movie theaters, over 110 restaurants, more than 800 stores and services, 58 entrances, and 325,000 light fixtures. It is also said to house the world's largest parking lot.

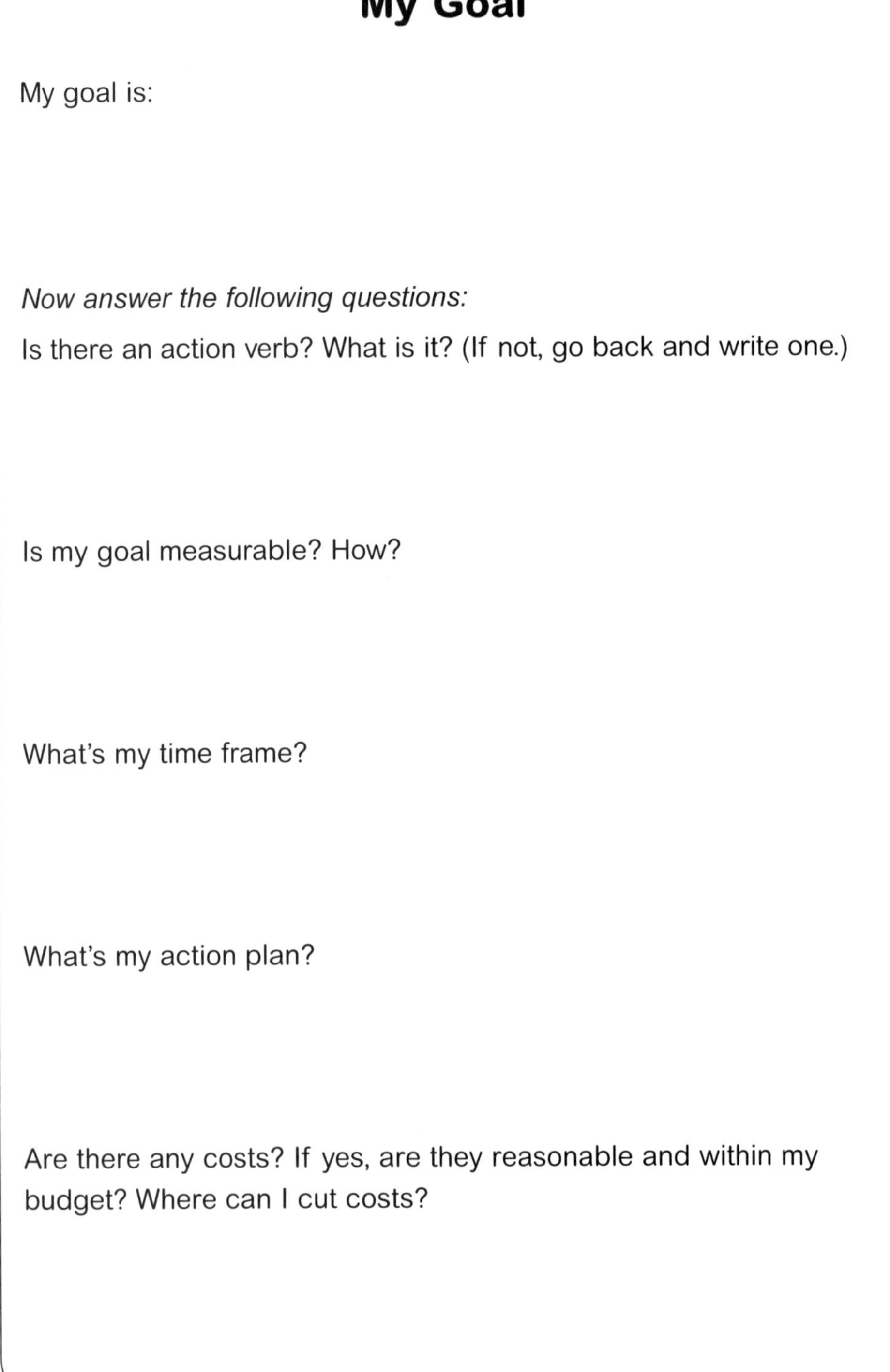

My Goal

My goal is:

Now answer the following questions:

Is there an action verb? What is it? (If not, go back and write one.)

Is my goal measurable? How?

What's my time frame?

What's my action plan?

Are there any costs? If yes, are they reasonable and within my budget? Where can I cut costs?

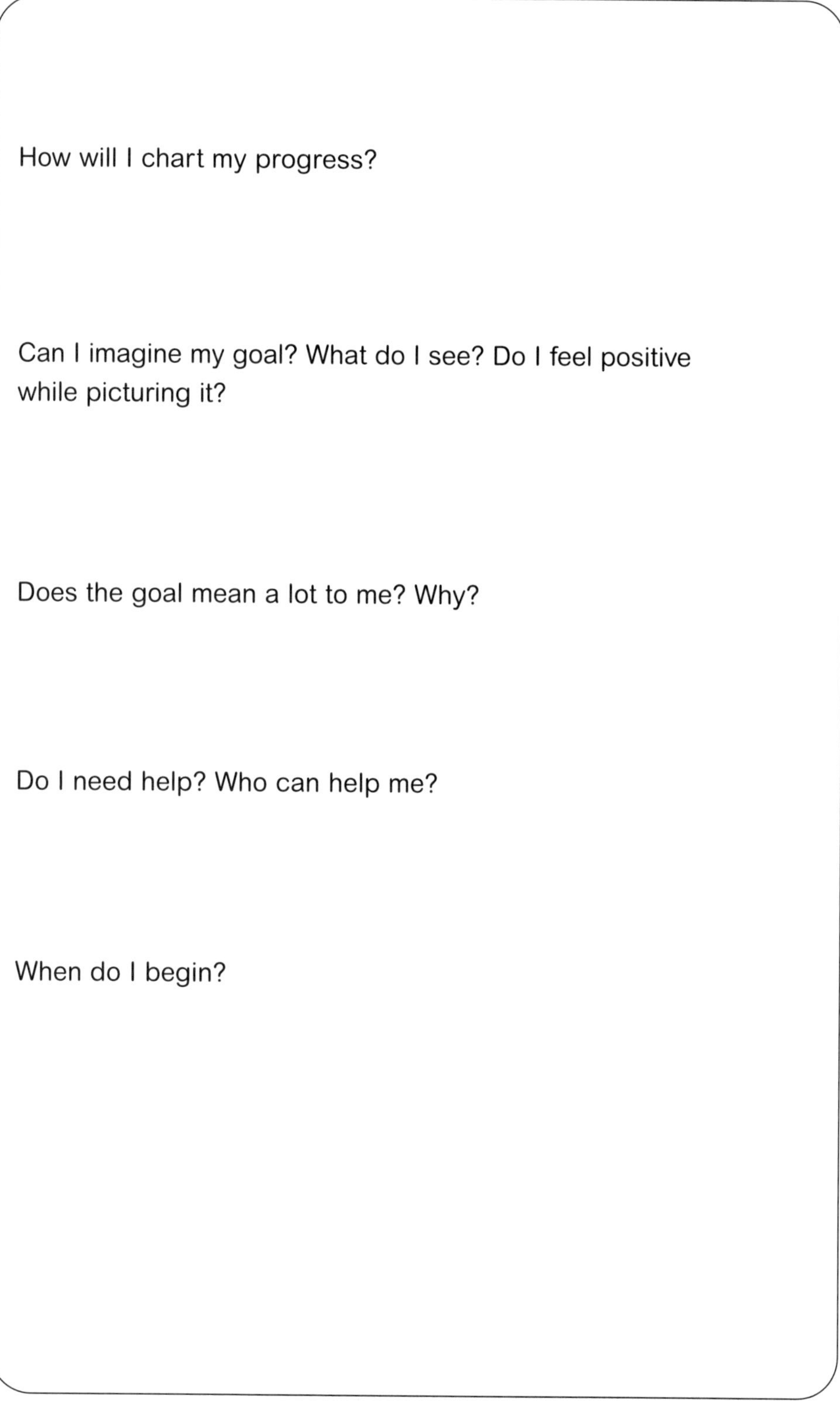

How will I chart my progress?

Can I imagine my goal? What do I see? Do I feel positive while picturing it?

Does the goal mean a lot to me? Why?

Do I need help? Who can help me?

When do I begin?

11 *Worthy* Walks

*W*alking has many personal benefits: It improves your health and self-esteem, brightens your social life, and adds purpose to your day. But walking can also benefit others, if you join in some of the many fund-raising activities in your area. Here's just a sampling of some of the worthy causes supported by walkers. Learn about what's happening in your community and see how you can get involved.

- **March for Parks,** an annual Earth Day event, is the nation's largest walking event for parks and open spaces. Sponsored by the National Parks and Conservation Association, it raises money to repair and build community parks, trails, and public walking space.

- **Dogs Walk** is the annual American Cancer Society's walk-athon for walkers with or without a pet. The walk raises money for human and animal cancer.
- **The American Heart Walk** takes place in more than 1,000 cities each year. The event raises money for heart research and consumer education to help prevent heart disease and stroke. Those who have survived a heart attack, heart surgery, or stroke wear a red hat during the walk, celebrating their renewed health.
- **The March of Dimes WalkAmerica** is one of the largest walking events in the nation, involving more than 875,000 people. Money raised from this walking classic goes to help prevent birth defects.
- **Walk for the Cure** is an annual worldwide event that raises money on behalf of juvenile diabetes. In Canada, more than 50,000 walkers join the Shoppers Walk for the Cure in twenty-four cities.
- **Race for the Cure,** a national race and fitness walk, supports research, education, screening, and treatment for breast cancer. Breast cancer survivors and those who have lost a loved one to breast cancer are honored with special ribbons.
- **The MS Walk for Multiple Sclerosis** raises money in the fight against multiple sclerosis. Chicago walkers have gained fame for organizing the largest MS walk in the nation, generating more than a million dollars.
- **The annual Walk for Animals** is the world's largest "pet walk." Walkers raise money for the Animal Humane Society.